ENERGY MEDICINE

ENERGY MEDICINE

The Science and Mystery of Healing

JILL BLAKEWAY

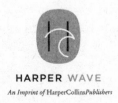

HARPER WAVE

An Imprint of HarperCollinsPublishers

HarperCollins books may be purchased for educational, business, or sales promotional use. For information, please email the Special Markets Department at SPsales@harpercollins.com.

FIRST EDITION

Designed by Bonni Leon-Berman

Library of Congress Cataloging-in-Publication Data has been applied for.

ISBN 978-0-06-269160-6

19 20 21 22 23 LSC 10 9 8 7 6 5 4 3 2 1

ALEX TIBERI WAS A HEALER AND A SCHOLAR.

*He was my first teacher and this book is
dedicated to his memory.*

CONTENTS

INTRODUCTION

In the 1840s, puerperal fever, or "childbed fever," a postpartum bacterial uterine infection, swept through one of two maternity clinics at the Vienna General Hospital in Austria. At the first clinic, the mortality rate among women giving birth was 10 percent; in the other, it was less than 4 percent. The two clinics admitted patients on alternate days. When women learned they'd gone into labor on a day reserved for the clinic rife with childbed fever, they would often drop to their knees, begging not to be admitted. Some women went so far as to stall long enough to give birth outside. These women—who'd given "street births" as this practice came to be known—remained eligible for child-care benefits, even without having to be admitted to the clinic. And, as it was later discovered, they also rarely contracted the childbed fever that was raging inside.

Ignaz Semmelweis, a Hungarian doctor who'd recently begun working at the first clinic, wondered what protected these women from such a highly contagious infection. After all, both clinics used almost all of the same techniques. The only difference: medical students worked in the first clinic whereas midwives worked in the second. After a meticulous process of elimination, Semmelweis concluded that he and the medical students carried "cadaverous particles" on their hands, whereas the midwives, who did not perform autopsies and had no contact with corpses, kept their hands free of such contamination. (As for the women who'd had street births, they'd managed to avoid infection by not having medical oversight during childbirth at all.)

Semmelweis subsequently ordered that doctors at the first clinic wash their hands with chlorinated lime water after performing autopsies and before examining patients. After the practice was instituted, the mortality rate at the first clinic dropped by an astounding 90 percent. Semmelweis then ordered the midwives at the second clinic to do the same—in addition to scrubbing their instruments in a chlorine solution. Again, this dramatically reduced the hospital's death rate.

Yet, despite clear evidence that Semmelweis's theory and practice saved lives, his colleagues, clinging to their well-established beliefs, refused to concede that these results were anything more than coincidence. After all, they couldn't see the cause of death: the microscopic bacteria. And, more important, Semmelweis's data didn't correspond with how they believed the body operated. The germ theory of disease had not yet been accepted in Vienna; diseases were attributed, at that time, to a variety of different and unrelated causes. Semmelweis's colleagues ridiculed him and eventually stopped following his guidelines. Soon after, Semmelweis lost his job. He spent the rest of his life fighting the medical community on this issue of sterilization and cleanliness, and at age forty-seven, this innovative thinker was committed to a mental asylum, where he died from sepsis.

The foundations of energy medicine are as ancient as history. In Egypt, a description of the laying on of hands, as a prompt to the body to relieve pain, was found in the Ebers Papyrus, one of the oldest preserved medical documents, dated 1550 BC. Pythagoras, the Greek philosopher and physician, considered healing his greatest calling and considered the pneuma, literally meaning "breath," to be the spirit. In Ayurveda, a health system developed thousands of years ago in India, the life-giving force is referred to as "prana"; in Judeo-Christian belief systems, it is called the "breath of life." And in traditional Chinese medicine (TCM), which is what I have practiced for twenty years, the animating force that plays an essential role in maintaining and restoring health is called "qi." In this way, spirituality, philosophy, and science were once intertwined, making up an essential part of our history, but we have since strayed considerably from this notion. I often wonder if one day we'll look back on energy healing and shake our heads in disbelief, as we do with the story of Semmelweis, wondering why any of us resisted an approach that offers such benefits simply because it didn't fit into our prevailing medical model.

And yet I admit: I, myself, took my time in coming around to this view. My career began with an instinct to help others; it was as broad and naive as that. But as my work took form—after studying East Asian medicine in graduate school, I practiced acupuncture in hospice before starting my own practice in New York City—I came to recognize the profoundly interwoven nature of healing.

From the start, in my work as an acupuncturist, I was both humbled and intrigued by the way patients thrived under my care. It bolstered my faith that this ancient practice—administering thin needles to affect the flow of energy within the body—

offered such effective results. It also, however, raised a number of startling questions. Most essentially: Why was it that this manipulation of energy was so beneficial? Was I simply acting as a placebo? Or was I some kind of conduit, as I sometimes curiously felt, with energy coming through me when I worked?

Chinese philosophy posits that a vital energy, what is called qi, surrounds and courses through our bodies to support life. It holds the body's innate intelligence, the intangible yet measurable way we maintain what's known as "homeostasis," or the body's ability to regulate its internal environment to create good health. But qi is also understood to be part of a larger pattern, a grand energy field, through which we are all interrelated.

As I became more adept at my work, I had the sense that something I couldn't see was influencing what was happening—not unlike, perhaps, the intuition Dr. Semmelweis felt in his clinic. I suspected that the needles and herbs (which I prescribe to supplement the acupuncture) were only part of what was helping my patients. And, increasingly, I felt an undeniable sensation when I practiced. Physically, it felt as if someone were pouring tonic water down my spine; mentally, it came across as an acute instinct that I was drawing energy from outside and channeling it for my patients.

I was captivated by this notion, but I was also afraid of it, impatient with it, wary of its validity. I was conscious of, and self-conscious about, the energy healing field being rife with—to put a fine point on it—quackery. While TCM practitioners like me are licensed and held to a specific standard both medically and ethically, there are no minimum standards for most other types of energy work, which makes this a precarious landscape to enter, with fellow practitioners who can hang a shingle and ask clients to simply have faith in what they do. The last thing I wanted to give people—including myself—was false hope. I never want to overpromise or underdeliver. (My policy, I should also say, has always been to recommend, and in some instances require, that my patients confer with the appropriate medical doctors in conjunction with my treatments.) But I also had the strong impulse to further explore this ancient medical system that sought to unify the physical and the energetic and to understand it within the worlds of science and spirituality and philosophy today.

As someone who methodically charts her own progress, I wasn't able to just accept that an enigmatic mix of needles and invisible energy fields served my patients so well. I wanted to know why. I also fervently wanted to explain me to me. So I pursued a variety of knowledgeable and dynamic specialists—healers, academics, doctors, scientists, and researchers on the cutting edge of energy medicine—and I found that they were all working from remarkably, and reassuringly, similar and interconnecting theories.

Moving from the scientific to the mystical and back again, this book has been both a deeply personal project and a professional inquiry. It is as important for me to take an unflinching look at what I may be experiencing as a healer as it is to measure the changes that arise from energy interventions, and to validate them with evidence-based research.

As such, over the last few years, I've studied the research of the former dean of engineering at Princeton University Robert Jahn, cofounder of the Princeton Engineering Anomalies Research (PEAR) lab, which developed its own experimental agenda for investigating collective consciousness and its effects on us. I was counseled on spirituality and healing by Neale Donald Walsch, the bestselling author of the series Conversations with God. In Japan I visited the healer Hiroyuki Abe, who applies energy to acupuncture points—without using needles. I asked a psychophysiologist to measure what happens in my body when I'm working with a patient, published research on energy medicine in the *Journal of Alternative and Complementary Medicine*, and consulted a British MD with an interesting take on how the acupuncture meridians work. I also spent time with William Bengston, PhD, author of *The Energy Cure: Unraveling the Mystery of Hands-On Healing*, who is both a healer and a scientist. Dr. Bengston trained a team of skeptical colleagues to use hands-on healing with lab mice who had been given injections that induced mammary cancer. The result? Dr. Bengston and his teams cured the mice time and again, in every experiment.

This book is an account of what I've come to know about the most dependable and impressive means of harnessing healing energy and how we can all make this powerful force work for us. I hope that readers will not only come away with an understanding of what healing energy is, but genuinely trust it and feel encouraged to explore their own needs in a more informed way. And, as I believe everyone has an innate ability to tap into healing energy within themselves and in the world around them, I have included exercises throughout the book to help readers draw on their own capacities.

While Chinese medicine will always be my foundation and focus, the work I do now is very different from when I first began my career—it is the result of various disciplines that span many cultures and belief systems. And, as I'd hoped, my patients are better for it. More unexpectedly, however, this search has allowed me an unwavering faith that what cannot be explained, the bit of mystery that will always lie just out of reach, may be attuned to our needs.

ENERGY MEDICINE

1

AT MY FINGERTIPS

The first acupuncture patient I ever worked with on my own was a woman who had broken both of her legs. She had visited a fire station with her women's group and had been encouraged, ill-advisedly as it turned out, to slide down the fire pole. When I met her, she was still walking with two canes—a full year after her accident.

I was just beginning my third year of a four-year master's degree in acupuncture and Chinese medicine in San Diego, California, and a long way from my native Britain. Before treating this woman, I'd only ever performed acupuncture on a patient as an assistant to a more senior student; before that, I'd practiced on sewn bags of rice. This was my first day working as an acupuncturist and herbalist in the school's clinic, and though I did have a supervisor, he was also watching a number of other students, all of us practicing acupuncture unaccompanied for the first time.

In the treatment room, the woman looked at me expectantly

and handed over a set of X-rays from her doctor. I held them up to the light and tried to at least *appear* confident as I attempted to decipher what exactly I was viewing. At that moment my supervisor popped his head around the door to check on me; he strode across the room to turn the X-rays right side up in my hands. "Just do a basic treatment," he told me quietly.

I forged ahead. I asked the woman to put on a gown and lie down on the small table. When she was ready, I dutifully began putting needles in a selection of basic acupuncture points to address her pain. The woman was completely still and silent throughout. Honestly, I had no sense as to whether anything I was doing was having any effect at all. The session seemed rather unremarkable—disappointingly so—until the end. What happened next will sound too good to be true, but bear with me: the point of this story is that it is easy to attribute recoveries we don't understand to the miraculous when, in fact, they are really just recoveries we don't understand.

After I had removed the last needle and whispered a quiet "Thank you" to indicate the treatment was over, the woman opened her eyes and said, "That felt amazing!" She sat upright from the table and declared, "I'm going to try walking without my canes." And that she did. She walked slowly round the room. I felt as if we were on a daytime talk show, the whole thing felt so surreal. I briefly wondered if this was some kind of test or prank that the teachers pulled on all first-timers.

But there she was, this woman who'd hobbled in only an hour ago, strolling out of the office. She even left her canes behind, propped up against the wall. I carried them out to the parking lot, where she was getting into her car. When I caught up to her, she offered me a curt and practical thank-you; I suppose she'd expected this much from an acupuncture session. I handed her the canes, my head still spinning, and thanked her back.

"What on earth did you do?" asked my supervisor when I returned. I had no idea. But it was immediately clear to me that, tempting as it was, I couldn't take credit. For a start, I wasn't sure that the patient's sudden impulse to walk, although dramatic, was all that miraculous. After a year of using canes, there was bound to come a time when she felt confident enough to discard them. Perhaps the acupuncture had given her sufficient pain relief that she felt as if this was the right day to try. It was also possible I'd played the role of a placebo, offering the psychological reassurance this woman needed to get up on her feet (quite literally).

Regardless, this experience was a pivotal one because it made me see that people can heal in astonishing ways. And I felt for the first time how deeply gratifying it is to guide people toward better health—even if I'm not entirely clear on *how* the healing has taken place. I felt not only a profound sense of purpose when I helped to relieve my patient's suffering but also a sense of inevitability—or, put more dramatically, fate. I knew on that day that this was what I was meant to do. This woman with the two broken legs and her striking response to treatment—be it the consequence of acupuncture or placebo or a more expansive energy or, as I now believe, some combination of the three—set me on a path. I began to understand with more nuance and depth that healing isn't magic, but rather a complicated interplay between circumstance, skill, and the body's own energy field, or what the Chinese refer to as qi.

. . .

The Chinese were not alone in identifying an animating force that plays an essential role in maintaining and restoring good health. In fact, most major cultural traditions identify a vital energy that governs physical and mental processes and provides all living beings with a blueprint for health and abundance.

What these ancient traditions observed more generally is that life has two aspects: matter and energy. They viewed the body as matter and identified its vital force—variously called pneuma, prana, or breath—as energy.

Of course, philosophers and Western scientists, too, are not strangers to the quest to understand what animates us. The Greek philosopher Aristotle actually coined the term *"enérgeia,"* which is Greek for energy, though it doesn't directly translate in English. Aristotle, himself, found it difficult to define what he meant by the word, as he used it to convey a variety of ideas, one of which is related to intention,[1] a desire to make manifest the decisions of the mind. In the seventeenth century, "energy" was first used in English to refer to "power," and in the nineteenth century it took on its more scientific meaning as a property that must be transferred to an object to perform work or to generate heat. In 1905, Albert Einstein offered a new way of looking at the relationship between energy and matter when he published a paper containing the famous equation $E=MC^2$—E being, of course, energy, M being mass (which is how we measure matter), and C^2, from the Latin word *"celeritas,"* meaning "quickness," referring to the speed of light.

Scientists had considered energy to be a property of matter before this, but Einstein's theory proposed that matter and energy are interrelated and that simply by having mass, matter possesses an inherent amount of energy. In those rare instances in which matter is totally converted into energy, Einstein's equation helps us calculate how much energy will be produced.

The idea that matter can be turned into energy may sound esoteric, but it's a principle with which we are all familiar. It's what happens when we burn wood in order to generate heat. It led to the development of the atomic bomb. But is the reverse true? Is matter simply energy condensed? The Big Bang would suggest that it is; this theory has energy converting into matter as the universe came into being. However, this is very challenging to prove in a practical way thanks to the C^2 part of Einstein's equation—the speed of light squared. Creating enough velocity—and consequently enough energy—to re-create such a phenomenon was considered an impossible task.

Until, that is, in 2012, when scientists at the European Organization for Nuclear Research (known as CERN, for Conseil Européenne pour la Recherche Nucléaire), the laboratory for particle physics near Geneva, were able to successfully create the Higgs particle, sometimes referred to as the God particle.[2] In order to do this, two particles—traveling an almost seventeen-mile ring from opposite directions—were collided at fantastically high energies. This collision took place in CERN's Large Hadron Collider—the world's most powerful particle accelerator—which took thirty years to build, cost $6.4 billion, and literally spans two countries (in order to get around it, scientists bike its perimeters, which stretch between France and Switzerland).

The creation of the Higgs particle was a tremendous success; however, it came with a caveat: the experiment had required a small amount of matter to initiate the process, which meant that it hadn't conclusively established that energy can be converted into matter. Until 2014, that is, when a group of physicists from Imperial College London and Germany's Max Planck Institute for Nuclear Physics offered an elegant solution.[3] They proved mathematically that two light particles (known as photons) could be collided to create matter.[4]

According to the Judeo-Christian belief system, on the first day of creation, God said, "Let there be light." In this way, when transforming pure energy into matter, science, as it turns out, is aligned with spirituality.

The Taoist version of the creation story, as it is known in Chinese philosophy, begins with nothingness, from which duality arises. This duality—held within the idea of qi or "life energy"—is composed of opposing, but interconnected, concepts: yin and yang. One cannot exist without the other. They complement each other in the world, forming a whole. Cold is yin and would not exist without comparison to heat, which is yang. Daytime belongs to yang; nighttime is yin. However, in medicine, yin refers to matter or, more specifically, the body—our bones, organs, muscles, blood vessels. Yang describes our circulating life force, or, as I think of it, our body's intelligence. Yin and Yang are in dynamic balance within us. Yin can turn into yang; yang can turn into yin. When one is excessive, the other is diminished and vice versa; the relationship is always changing. TCM advises that there can be both external (something outside of us such as germs or poor diet) and internal (which includes emotions as well as our genes) influences that affect yin and yang.

Chinese medicine also, thousands of years ago, accounted for the consequence of the external on the internal—not unlike today's epigenetic research that suggests, for example, that the food we consume[5] may cause damaging modifications to our DNA. Likewise, the teachings of TCM suggest that unexpressed or extreme negative emotion from our life experiences can cause illness, creating stagnation or blockage. This is where energy medicine comes in: it helps to reestablish a flow of energy, bringing yin and yang back into balance and revitalizing qi.

Chinese philosophy also posits that our personal energy field is part of a greater energy field known as the Tao. The Tao, which is said to be so boundless it defies description, is the natural order of the universe and the container for all of our experiences as human beings. The sixth-century Chinese text Hsin-Hsin Ming (which translates to "Faith-Mind Verses") describes the Tao as "like vast space where nothing is lacking and nothing is in excess."[6]

This sounds rather peaceful, doesn't it? And it would be, except that every feeling we experience, every thought we have, every action we take, causes a ripple of disturbance in the Tao, like a pebble thrown into a smooth lake. And those ripples affect not just ourselves, but everyone, because as the Hsin-Hsin Ming reminds us, we are, as people, "not two"—that is, "nothing is separate, nothing is excluded"[7] from the Tao. In other words, all living beings are interrelated.

This interconnectedness, through the Tao, our shared container—what is sometimes referred to as the "universal energy field" in energy medicine—might also reflect on one of the strangest discoveries in quantum physics: the concept of nonlocality. Scientists have found that when subatomic particles (particles that are smaller than an atom) are separated, they behave as if time and space don't exist and communicate with each other instantaneously. If one particle makes a "decision," the other knows about it immediately and reacts. For example, when a laser is shone through a certain type of crystal, the light particles split and become entangled even though separated by a large distance; in these circumstances, it has been observed that one of the paired photons spins upward whereas its partner spins downward. This dynamic balance is strikingly reminiscent of the relationship the Chinese observed between yin and yang. Furthermore, this communication between particles happens at a speed that is at least ten thousand times the speed of light and likely instantaneous. This puzzled Einstein, who believed he had proven that the speed of light was the maximum speed for anything in the universe. He dismissively referred to this phenomenon as "spooky actions at a distance,"[8] but in the quantum world it is now an established fact that these "spooky actions" are real. In addition, once particles become entangled, they are permanently enmeshed in a way that makes them behave as if they are a single entity—even when they are far apart.

Physicists insist that, because human beings are made up of billions of atoms, we are more likely to respond to statistical laws than quantum ones. But what if they're wrong? What if we are interconnected in ways that we are yet to understand? What if we are connected and influenced by a vast energy field that is the same phenomenon that the ancient Chinese called the Tao?

. . .

I believe that humans might be similarly "entangled," connecting us within a larger energy field. Most often this thought occurs to me while I am treating a patient. Much of the information I get about a patient comes from the standard procedures of TCM—taking the pulse, looking at the tongue (there is an entire system of diagnosis based on the shape and coating), getting a person's full medical history—but there are also times when what I glean comes to me in other ways. Recently, I met with a longtime patient of mine, a young man named Alex I've been seeing for over a decade. He had been diagnosed with pneumonia by his doctor and, although he'd taken a full round of antibiotics, was still suffering from a terrible cough and fatigue. Both of these symptoms were enough for me to recommend he see his doctor again. He should have felt some improvement from the medication and he was clearly still unwell. Experience has taught me that I can sometimes feel areas of stagnation in a person's energy field by moving my hands a few inches above their body and looking for areas that feel denser and harder to move my hands over. I found one such area in Alex's right lung and kept my hand still as I tried to understand what I was feeling. It was, I realized, a feeling of foreboding. I must have looked worried because Alex took notice. "Oh, I forgot to mention it, but that is a spot that feels a bit painful," he said. He described the discomfort as "a deep ache." He went on to say that he was doing his best to rest and recover because he was scheduled to travel to Europe the following day for work.

"You can't take a flight tomorrow without seeing your doctor first," I said with some force. I surprised even myself with the sharpness of my tone. I'd felt dread as I said it, but I couldn't name why exactly, and soon, I was doubling back, trying not to sound so dire. "I mean I think it's important that you tell your doctor that the round of antibiotics didn't help," I said, trying to ground my response in reason. "And you should have him take a look at your lungs; you shouldn't still be experiencing pain." I'd known to give him that advice medically, yes, but my feeling of unease was also coming to me as strong intuition. There was a terrific doctor whom I worked with from time to time when I was based in a hospice; he used to say, "If your patient is in a coma and you feel uncomfortable, they're probably feeling uncomfortable too." His point being that we can pick things up intuitively from our patients. That may be, in part, because our experience as practitioners has become so deeply ingrained, sometimes our expertise can feel like second nature. And yet I believe there is something else that happens, too, as it did with Alex. My fear felt so disproportionate and overwhelming in that moment, I believe I wasn't just picking up information from Alex himself but also from the field in which we are all connected.

That night, Alex's wife called me from the hospital, where they were keeping Alex overnight for observation. He'd dutifully visited his doctor that afternoon and discovered that he had been misdiagnosed with pneumonia. Instead his symptoms were caused by a pulmonary embolism, a blockage in one of the arteries of his lungs. His doctor explained to him that he could have had a heart attack, from the restriction of blood flow in his lungs, if he'd gotten on a plane.

I do understand how odd a story like this can sound to people. In fact, I, myself, often wonder if some of these things really happen in the way that I remember them. Over time, I can poke holes in these stories, small punctures that let the air out of them, flattening them into more rational thought. Yet each time I have an experience like this—and something inevitably occurs to revive my sense of the extraordinary—it takes me another step toward understanding the web of energetic connections that underpins our ability to heal ourselves as well as each other. So, even though I was—and always will be—questioning my experiences and seeking explanations, I had also begun to simultaneously develop faith in myself as a conduit for healing energy as well as in the universe as the source.

Though I do strongly believe that anyone can develop their healing energy, I have also come to understand that there are certain experiences that make some of us more attuned to it than others. One commonality among people who are highly attuned to the energy around them is that many have experienced trauma or endured acute stress at a young age. Certainly, this is true for me.

My mother was a troubled and unhappy woman. Brought up in an abusive household, she sought escape by marrying my father at the age of twenty; at twenty-one, she had a small baby—me—and then another child, my brother, three years later. Despite her intention to escape abuse by building her own family, she found she was now facing a new set of challenges.

My father was a professional motorcycle racer and well known in England at the time, as he was often on television. He was sponsored by a major motorcycle manufacturer and was on the road constantly, traveling to compete all over Europe. One of my earliest memories is accompanying my father for a lap of honor—

seated with him on his motorbike—in celebration of his winning a motocross event. The noise of the bikes and the enthusiastic roar of the crowd proved too much for my two-year-old self. I remember wailing until I was handed back to my mother to be comforted.

I wasn't the only one overwhelmed by my father's success: my mother, barely out of her teens, with two small children, was struggling to cope, especially with her husband so often away. My father's mother lived next door; instead of offering an extra set of hands, however, she was a constant source of criticism, bordering on contempt. My grandmother had had a privileged upbringing and resented my father marrying, as she saw it, beneath him. Despite being a lay preacher in the Methodist church, she never missed an opportunity to judge my mother. Young, vulnerable, and feeling in over her head, my mother began to implode.

She struggled with mental illness during a period of time when it was still lurking in the shadows of awareness. There wasn't the psychiatric care or medication that is available now. Had my mother been tended to properly, I believe she would have been medicated for her severe depression as well as her paranoid, angry outbursts. Perhaps she would have been able to find balance early enough so as not to have to go through so much of the anguish and explosions of temper that she suffered in those years. But instead she was given bad advice and, ultimately, underwent repeated electric shock treatments. This left her flat and emotionless for months at a time, and resulted in permanent memory loss and a sense of disconnection.

I understand now that she was trying to mother two small children under psychologically untenable conditions. But, from my young perspective, I saw a mother who was unpredictable and terrifying: one moment she was lovely, and the next she was screaming and violent. My thoughts tacked between *she's going to kill me* and *she's not going to kill me* almost minute to minute as I vacillated between fear and love. I was three years older than my brother and felt responsible for keeping us both safe. In order to do so, I had to read my mother's moods with a scrutiny that felt as if our lives depended on it. I grew hypervigilant, constantly scanning the adults around me for nonverbal cues. In particular, I would study my mother's face and body, looking for the steely set of her jaw or swiftness of her gestures that hinted at a storm brewing within. One of my most vivid memories from childhood is of an afternoon in which I assumed a primal fetal position on the floor, my brother curled within me, my arms cocooned around our heads, as she lashed out, attacking us in a dark moment of emotional disturbance.

But my childhood suffering, I believe, also helped me to cultivate—instinctively if not consciously—the dynamic awareness necessary for energy healing. Many years later, as I was seeking to learn more about my practice, I encountered a woman who has taught many of the best-known psychic mediums. She explained that trauma is often linked to psychic ability as well: people with volatile backgrounds are more likely to have nurtured a sense of premonition, and they are better at picking up information from the energy field.

This idea was affirmed for me when, in the aftermath of the 9/11 terrorist attack on the World Trade Center in 2001, I found myself treating a team of FBI intelligence officers in New York who were in extreme distress; they were second-guessing themselves, literally worrying themselves sick that they had missed a crucial piece of information, the clue that might have helped to prevent the attack. What was fascinating in treating them—and this was universally true among them—is that they felt my acupuncture needles *before* they went in. Lying on the table, eyes closed or staring upward at the ceiling, each one reliably flinched just before I'd place the needle in their arms or legs or feet. Some might say these officers were on such high alert they were probably flinching when anything came near them. In Chinese medicine, however, we'd say that they'd moved their qi—or, more accurately, their *wei qi* (which is translated as defensive energy) outside their body in order to be on a perpetual high alert. Already devastated by the tragedy that had just occurred, they were now spending their days combing through intelligence to determine if another attack was about to happen. As a result, they were unusually receptive to the energy around them—to the point of being able to physically feel something in advance of it actually touching them.

Despite my difficult childhood, I consider myself to have had a proper British upbringing. My grandparents paid for me to go to expensive private schools, where I'd try to fit in and hide what was happening at home. The urge to belong—and the shame I felt at being different—meant that I was passionately drawn to a conventional life. The worst thing I could have imagined was being perceived as weird. I still sometimes have to fight the instinct that being an energy healer is too far out of the realm of an acceptable path for me, that I was actually meant to live in a country house in my native Yorkshire with an AGA stove and a pile of kids and dogs, quietly allowing my extrasensory perceptions to play out within the safe confines of tradition.

I'd beelined for a traditional life after college, first working as a money broker, then getting engaged at twenty-five years old—to my boss, which perhaps did not entirely line up with my pursuit of convention—and later becoming a fund-raiser for a charitable trust founded by members of the British royal family. But when, three years later, I separated from my husband just a few weeks after giving birth to my daughter (marrying the boss, as it turned out, had been a bad idea), I found myself in such a tailspin that I vaulted myself into an entirely new, decidedly less conventional existence.

I moved, with my newborn daughter in tow, to Key West, Florida, to work for a mail-order catalog company. The catalog offered an array of paraphernalia marketed toward the gay community. I was writing catalog copy, mostly—which I could do anywhere—so I would take a laptop (a first-generation Apple laptop, more like carrying along a microwave), a beach umbrella, a folding chair, and baby Emma to the beach, where we would sit for hours while I did my "job."

But it was also in Key West that I became fascinated by acupuncture. I went to see a local practitioner recommended to me by a woman in a health-food store when I'd complained of an array of minor but irritating health problems. I was utterly taken by the ritual—the slender needles urging my energy into balance— and the swift recovery I made afterward. I was curious to learn more about this phenomenal technique, and so I asked the practitioner if I might sit in on some of his appointments with his patients' permission.

I had come to Key West in the early 1990s, a bewildered, newly single mother, just as so many gay young men were also arriving on the island, exiling themselves from families and communities where they'd been ostracized for having AIDS. These were some of the most incredible people I'd ever met, brilliant and warm and full of promise—it was so difficult to realize that they were going to have to leave the earth sooner than they should. Many of them became patients of the acupuncturist I was shadowing, and I observed as he treated them. He was an excellent practitioner and a tenacious advocate for the gay community. I watched him care for these men, buoying them as they grew ever thinner and paler; I saw the relief that flooded their faces when he was able to lift their pain and offer them at least a little more time in bodies that weren't completely betraying them. I also saw a possibility for myself. I felt a distant sense of calling; I wanted to provide the same kind of release and support—I knew that much. I also knew that I wanted to learn Eastern medicine in conjunction with Western medicine. I wanted to be part of a medical community that was rigorous about, and respectful of, both worlds. So I applied to the Pacific College of Oriental Medicine in San Diego, California—one of the best schools in the US to study East Asian medicine—and was accepted into their master of science program.

I wasn't sure what to expect, but Eastern medicine turned out to be an absorbing field of study. Acupuncturists are licensed in most American states and are therefore regulated as part of the broader medical community, which means they are required to take many of the same courses as any other medical student— classes such as anatomy (with cadavers), chemistry, biophysics, pathophysiology, pharmacology, and research methods. These classes are interwoven with courses on Chinese philosophy and its impact on diagnosis and treatment. As I threw myself into learning herbalism and acupoint location, while also immersing myself in biology and physics, I had a revelation: the dichotomy, and conflict, being expressed in my studies was the same one scientists have been wrestling with for hundreds of years—that is, the relationship between matter and energy.

Western medicine is rooted in the work of Sir Isaac Newton, the seventeenth-century physicist who is considered to be the father of modern science. Newton saw the universe as a massive mechanical system in which space and time are absolute.[9] And it's from this basis that doctors are taught to think of the body as a machine, controlled by the brain via the nervous system and made up of other systems with various functions that can therefore malfunction. Eastern thought, however, has always encompassed the idea that our essence is energetic—that we are, in effect, energy condensed.

By my fourth year at acupuncture school, I was considered skilled enough to work under supervision in a hospital setting. I was sent to work at a local hospice and found it a great fit for my intuitive and healing skills; it also introduced me to the profound nature of energy work as well as how I might play a role within it.

Here, I spent my time with people of all ages and illnesses; the only thing that they had in common—aside from the singular daring each one of them displayed in finally letting go—was that they were going to have to let go. In order to be an effective practitioner, I quickly realized, I'd need to move my ego out of the way and give up my notion of healing these patients.

Within months of starting, I was summoned to treat an Irish man in his early forties—only a decade or so older than me—who was dying of cancer and in quite a lot of pain. I felt a special pang of sympathy for him because he was also an expat, far from home and without his family. I went to him right away and began to massage his feet and legs. He seemed only mildly relieved. I eagerly flipped through the options in my mind and had what I thought was a flash of inspiration: I would try a Chinese massage technique I'd recently learned called Pok, which required me rolling this man onto his front, cupping my hand and hitting his back in order for him to expel phlegm from his lungs. He coughed mightily. I rolled him onto his back again. He said nothing; I massaged his temples lightly.

"Is there anything else I can do for you?" I asked.

He nodded politely. "Yes," he replied, "please stop."

I took my hands away from his head.

He smiled and said, "Would you mind listening to me?" and nodded toward the chair next to him. I sat. He took my hand and began telling me about the small town he was from in Ireland. He described the farm he grew up on, how hard his dad had worked, the various characters of his many brothers and sisters, and the little lane he walked down to school. As he told his stories, he grew more animated and colorful, both in body and spirit, and I was happy to see him appear so full of life. I'd been told that his greatest wish was to go home to Ireland to die. When I left him that afternoon, I expected he'd have to die at hospice. Instead, over the next few days, he rallied and, despite still being very sick, his doctors considered him well enough to travel. He was able to fly back to Ireland, where he passed in his family's home.

Looking back, I realized that before he'd courteously asked me to stop, I'd treated that lovely Irishman like a rag doll, turning him this way and that, in an effort to relieve him but also with the hope that I might achieve admirable results. Had I let go of my ego, I'd have known that my remedies weren't necessary. He knew that; he was simply being kind enough to let me go through the motions. I realized then that if I esteemed myself for fixing people, or making them better, my work would be a frustrating and overwhelming experience. But if I could discern how I might *actually* be of service to my patients, how I could support their wishes and make their end-of-life experiences as peaceful as possible, it would be a meaningful one.

The inevitability of these hospice patients' outcomes, while sorrowful, also educated me in the dynamic energy of death. We tend to think of this passage as an end, even, in explicit medical terms, as a failure (heart failure, liver failure, kidney failure), but in my hospice work, I came to see it as a transformation. In Taoism, the process of death itself is described as "*shijie*," or "release from the corpse." Likewise, the first law of thermodynamics, a physicist will explain, asserts that the total energy of an isolated system is constant; energy can be transformed from one form to another but cannot be created or destroyed. And I have come to believe this is true in relation to personal energy too: at death, the energy leaves the body, but it is not gone; it assimilates back into the larger energetic field in which we all exist.

In Chinese medicine, the energy of a dying person is understood to be dynamic because the yin (substance and form, such as the body) and the yang (the energetic part of an individual) are separating. Yin and yang are in constant relation with each other throughout our lives, creating balance and imbalance. At death, however, as the yin comes to an end, the yang becomes chaotic and unanchored, creating an extremely active energy field. In my work with hospice patients, I found that acupuncture, which can positively affect the personal energy field, helped to bring order to this chaos; it provided relief, albeit temporarily, from the suffering my patients endured while trying to die.

As I became more experienced, and more comfortable, in helping people to navigate this intense uncoupling of yin and yang, I discovered that, if I placed my hand about three inches from the tops of their heads, I could feel their energy hitting my palm. It felt like a distinct pulse, almost a tap, and from this, I began to piece together my own interpretation of the energetic anatomy—that is, an understanding of how energy flows in the body. I drew from my own experience as well as culled from various cultures and philosophies. In acupuncture school, I'd been taught about energy channels (sometimes referred to as meridians), a kind of highway that can be mapped within the body along which the acupuncture points exist. But, in hospice, as I felt the patients' energy in various locations, I blended the principles of TCM's energetic map with the notion of chakras. Chakras are a concept with roots in a variety of Eastern philosophies; they are believed to be the psychic energy centers of the subtle body, or the energetic body. In Sanskrit, the term actually means "wheel," and each one is found in an area of the body that contains bundles of nerves and major organs. I came to believe the chakras are the locations where energy flows in and out of the body, while the channel system explains the way energy moves through the body. So, when I was holding my hand at the head of a dying person, feeling a tapping against my palm, this was their energy leaving through the crown chakra. Over time, I became practiced enough to be able to determine how close people were to death based on how intensely their energy was hitting my hand.

Ironically, while I was working in hospice supporting patients as they died, my own mother's life was ending after a four-year battle with breast cancer. When my father called me and said that it looked as if my mother's death was imminent, I flew to Scotland, where my parents were living. I walked into the bedroom, holding my eight-year-old daughter's hand, and saw that my mother had already moved past the most difficult stage: she was surrendering to death. I'd spent much of my adult life trying to lift my mother up after our difficult time together in my childhood. I'd taken her to medical doctors, psychiatrists, and self-esteem workshops—and, of course, I'd treated her with acupuncture too. Though she grew more stable, she was never someone I'd describe as happy. Still, we had managed to forge a durable relationship. I'd grown up enough to reasonably let go of my resentments and regrets about my childhood; I knew that she had done what she could, given the circumstances. I was aware of how extreme the sacrifices of motherhood had been for her particularly—she'd had all of the ordinary burdens while also thrashing about within, trying to keep hold of her mind. Now, here with her at the end of her life, I was also able to bring my knowledge from hospice to guide her. I sat down next to her. "I'm

here now, Mom," I whispered. She squeezed my hand. She had
been only intermittently conscious for days; I believe she'd been
waiting for me to arrive. We put on the classical guitar music that
she loved, opened the window and let a bit of sun and fresh air
into the room (not an easy feat in Scotland, where good weather
is a rarity), and I gave her a light acupuncture treatment to relieve
her discomfort. After seeing so many deaths in hospice—and the
instinctual defiance and struggle that come with this passage—I
was able to recognize the grace with which my mother was ac-
cepting her end. It was a pleasure, in a strange way, to see this
volatile woman experiencing such calm. I hadn't quite realized
how endeavoring to offer my mother the peace she ultimately
found on her deathbed had become the thrust of my adult life
until a friend recently remarked: "It's interesting, isn't it, after a
frightening childhood like yours, that you've made a living out of
trying to heal others by making them feel safe?"

I began my own acupuncture practice in New York City in 1999.
I was thirty-five years old, a devoted mother to my nine-year-old
daughter, and newly involved with a fellow acupuncturist named
Noah—who, in time, would become my husband. My office was
essentially a very small rented room within a suite of offices in a
building near Union Square. But my little business thrived from
the start. Within two years of starting my practice, I'd expanded
to four rooms and was seeing over a hundred patients a week
based primarily on word of mouth. Demand was high enough
that I had to start a waiting list.

One of my early clients, a man named Andrew, was a senior

executive for a financial institution and very successful in the stock market; he'd fly in by helicopter to see me every week to treat his back pain. A year into our working together, Andrew came in for an appointment, acting more solemn than usual. When we sat down to chat, as we always did before a session, he told me that he had been diagnosed with prostate cancer. But he had a dignified sense of optimism, and he was intent on regaining his health. At a certain point in our conversation, he looked at me and said: "I think we can turn this around together."

I was terrified. Since I'd started my practice, I had experimented occasionally with channeling energy through my hands and into the acupuncture needles when it felt right. I could not yet summon this energy on command, but at times, when I felt that it was there to be tapped, I would let it flow. Patients occasionally even remarked that they noticed something was different when I did. Some said they felt a charge, others felt warmth or tingling, and more than once patients referred to my "magnetic hands." But I had never taken on a life-threatening illness with a patient before—as an acupuncturist or otherwise. More important, I have never advised my patients to go it alone with acupuncture or any other healing medicine without the consult of a doctor; I am a firm believer in integrative medical partnerships.

But Andrew was prepared for this. He'd made an agreement with his doctors (never one to not be fully prepared, he'd been treated at Johns Hopkins and then sought a second opinion from Sloan Kettering): Andrew could take three months—his cancer was at a stage that his doctors felt would progress slowly and needed only be monitored during this time. We were to work together to see if he could reduce his Gleason score (the scale that doctors use to typify the severity of prostate cancer)—which had been diagnosed as 6.7—on his own. Though his Gleason score was on the higher side for a wait-and-see approach, his PSA (prostate-specific antigen) was low, which was unusual. Andrew wanted to get rid of his cancer, of course, but he was also resolute about not wanting to undergo the surgery that is advised with later stages of prostate cancer, which poses a risk of impotence, among other consequences.

So we crafted a collaborative regimen. I gave him weekly acupuncture treatments and worked out herbal preparations with practitioners more experienced than I was at the time. When I could, I brought healing energy to the fore in our sessions. It was a disconcerting transition for me; by turns, I was grateful and confused. *What am I doing?* I asked myself more than once. I had worked with people with cancer in hospice, but they were undeniably going to die. In this case, I was being asked to help someone in reversing the course of his illness. I took this as a grave responsibility, which made it impossible not to experience a healthy dose of self-doubt. But Andrew had almost more faith in me than I had in myself. We discussed the importance of taking a holistic approach when attempting a health transformation of this kind. I advised him to explore past traumas and conflicts in order to surface unresolved emotional suffering, which can create areas of stuck energy in a person's body; the lack of flow can make it difficult to turn the tide on one's health. Committed as ever, Andrew contacted family members he'd been avoiding rather than confronting emotional difficulties. He turned toward his Catholic church community for support as well as to reconnect with his sense of there being a mysterious force at work in the world. He focused on his diet and exercised regularly. Everything that I advised Andrew to do—the acupuncture, energy work, emotional healing, connection with spirit, healthy lifestyle—was designed to give him his best shot at recovery based on what I knew about the body's innate intelligence and its desire to energetically heal itself.

I also felt the strength of the energy come through me more vigorously than ever before. I've since learned that this happens when I am treating someone who is in dire need. I don't know whether this means the energy actually becomes more powerful or the person is more open to it—perhaps it is a bit of both. Whatever the case, the energy expressed itself in me with a distinct physical sensation: my back would straighten, and I would feel a kind of fizzy tingling throughout my body. It felt refreshing, as if I had tonic water rushing through my spine.

At the end of three months, Andrew consulted with his doctor, who gave him another biopsy. To both of our astonishment and relief, it showed that there was no longer any cancer. When he tried to tell his doctors that he believed that acupuncture, as well as the terrible-tasting Chinese herbs he'd had to drink at my behest, had helped to make the difference, they brushed this aside, preferring instead to explain that he'd been one of the lucky ones who'd gone through a "spontaneous remission." Either way, fifteen years later, Andrew is still healthy; the cancer has not come back.

This experience changed many things for me. To start, it gave me more confidence in my instincts and process. It was impossible to pull apart the strands of our collaboration—the energy healing, the acupuncture, his commitment, the psychological exploration, the support he received from his community—to know what had had the strongest effect, but I felt validated that our concerted effort had been worthwhile. More important, however, it helped me understand how much bigger the energy, and the work, is than I am. In hospice, I'd figured out how to put my own needs aside in order to create a direct path toward helping a patient, but I'd not quite realized that the healing power I offered wasn't actually coming from me. Working with Andrew made me profoundly aware that the energy I used to heal came from *outside of myself.* And I was becoming increasingly more sensitive to picking it up. As I continued to use energy in my practice, I started to grasp that, although the strength and duration of the energy changes was based on patients' needs, it invariably came from the same all-encompassing source: the universe.

YOU THE HEALER

Experiencing Energy

Understanding that your body is matter is easy. It's as simple as looking at your hands, but experiencing the energy that animates the body requires more subtlety. You can train yourself to feel your energy field with the following exercise. Experiencing your own energy field is the first step to connecting to other people's and using that connection to help them.

- Sit comfortably with your back straight. Spend a few minutes breathing deeply into your abdomen, allowing your mind to become quiet.

- Hold your hands out in front of you with the palms facing each other. Relax your hands so your fingers are slightly curled.
- Slowly bring your hands together until the palms are about two feet apart.
- Make small circular movements, with the palms facing each other. Feel the variations in sensation.
- Then separate your hands, palms still facing, and move them a little closer and farther from each other.
- Repeat this process several times, slowly bringing your hands together and apart.
- As you do it, pay close attention to your palms. Some of you may experience a sense of pressure between them, similar to magnets repelling each other. You may also experience warmth or a feeling of tingling or pulsing.
- Do this exercise for five minutes each day. As you finish the exercise, write down what you experienced and any feelings or thoughts you noticed.

Don't worry if you feel something different from what is described above. People experience this energy in different ways. And don't worry if you don't feel anything. I'm going to stick my neck out and make a prediction that if you continue to read and practice the exercises in this book you will experience this energy getting stronger by the time you reach the end.

2

THE SCIENCE
OF CONNECTION

Here is what we—Eastern medicine, Western medicine, science—
agree on: fields exist. A field, in this context, is an invisible region
that connects points in space. A variety of fields emanate from
an object. And, as a physicist will tell you, these fields extend
infinitely into space. The first person to suggest the notion of a
field was Isaac Newton. As the story goes, he conceived of gravity when he saw an apple fall from a tree and questioned the
force that would make this occur; in 1687, Newton published
Philosophiæ Naturalis Principia Mathematica,[1] in which he put
forth the concept of a gravitational field to explain the field of influence that an object with mass extends into space around itself,
producing an attractive force on another object or body.

After Newton, our understanding of fields continued to evolve,
with perhaps the biggest breakthrough arriving with a new awareness about how electricity and magnetism interact, forming what

we now call an electromagnetic field. This critical discovery, how-ever, required a fairly radical shift in mind-set, and, as with all radical shifts in mind-set, it took time. As such, our understanding of the electromagnetic field evolved over a series of scientific investigations spanning the lives of three men.

Michael Faraday, born in England in 1791 to a blacksmith and raised with little formal education, became, despite the odds, a respected and influential scientist. He discovered the chemical compound benzene and invented an early version of the Bunsen burner, but his most important contribution to science was establishing the notion of electromagnetism. Whereas classical, or Newtonian, physics was concerned with a set of laws that described motion under the influence of force, Faraday's concept was that "lines of flux"—or magnetic lines of force—emanate from charged bodies and magnets, creating an electromagnetic field. With this, we began to see a field as not just a way of calculating the force exerted on another object but also as an area through which energy can be transmitted more generally. Faraday also was the first to propose that fields extend infinitely. (Incidentally, the Faraday cage, an enclosure used to block out electromagnetic fields, invented by Faraday in 1836, is still widely used in experiments today.)

Like Dr. Ignaz Semmelweis, the pioneer of antisepsis in hospitals, however, Faraday was ridiculed by his contemporaries; not only did his Laws of Electromagnetic Induction involve hidden forces, but they also altered Newton's prevailing view of the universe. Faraday was shifting the focus of field theory from Newton's macro perspective, looking at the mechanics, to a micro perspective, which examined the transfer of energy at a microscopic level.

Though Faraday would not live to see it, the scientific community eventually came to accept his proposition.

In 1865, a Scottish mathematician named James Clerk Maxwell set out to express Faraday's theory in mathematical terms. Though Faraday was a brilliant scientist, he was not an agile mathematician; in fact, not one of his experiments involved advanced math. So Maxwell stepped in, putting forth a series of equations that demonstrated how electric and magnetic fields are generated by charges, currents, and the changes in each when they interact. One of the most critical components of Maxwell's work was his suggestion that the electromagnetic waves of a field move at the speed of light. Even light itself, Maxwell theorized, was an electromagnetic wave. His work not only legitimized Faraday's research but also helped to carry it into the future. To this day, Maxwell's equations are accepted as the basis of all modern theories of electromagnetic phenomena.

A little more than two decades later, a German physicist named Heinrich Hertz conclusively proved the existence of the electromagnetic field, rendering Faraday's "lines of flux" a confirmed phenomenon. To do this, Hertz designed a series of experiments[2] using an oscillator to conduct an electric current in a receiver loop placed several yards away that showed that a moving electric charge radiates electromagnetic waves. Hertz also measured Maxwell's waves, showing that their velocity was equal to the velocity of light. Electromagnetic waves are measured by their wavelength, energy, and frequency. "Frequency" refers to the number of times a wave oscillates within a particular time period. Today, we measure the frequency of alternating electric current, sound, and electromagnetic waves in a unit called a hertz, to honor Heinrich Hertz's groundbreaking work.

Together, these three men—Faraday, Maxwell, and Hertz—opened the door to revolutionary new areas of scientific knowledge. First came wireless telegraphy, which was used to transmit Morse code, and then X-ray, radio, television, radar, and the now-ubiquitous mobile phone.

Once Hertz established that both Faraday and Maxwell had been correct in claiming electromagnetic fields exist, scientists embraced the idea that the universe extends beyond the world we perceive with our senses. This set the stage for some of the most important discoveries of the twentieth century, including Einstein's special theory of relativity—which essentially proposes that space and time aren't separate entities—and the standard model of particle physics. It also changed the way scientists think about the physical world, prompting the arrival of quantum physics.

Quantum physics studies the ways matter and energy behave on the scale of atoms and subatomic particles and waves. Max Planck, a pioneer in this emerging world, won the Nobel Prize in physics in 1918 for his theory that electromagnetic energy is absorbed or emitted in discrete packets, otherwise known as quanta. Considered to be the father of quantum physics, Planck at times speaks about his discoveries in ways that echo the mystical. "As a man who has devoted his whole life to the most clearheaded science, to the study of matter, I can tell you as a result of my research about the atoms this much: There is no matter as such!"

he explained to an audience in Florence, Italy, in 1944. "All matter originates and exists only by virtue of a force which brings the particles of an atom to vibration and holds this most minute solar system of the atom together . . . We must assume behind this force the existence of a conscious and intelligent Mind. This Mind is the matrix of all matter."[3]

This "matrix," in quantum physics, is called the zero point field (ZPF).[4] Imagine you are on a beach watching two pebbles rolling in unison as they are buffeted by waves. If you didn't understand the role of the ocean in making them move, you would be forgiven for thinking that one pebble was communicating with the other—that, as Einstein would say, you were watching "spooky actions at a distance." The ocean, in this case, would be the zero point field, the invisible field generated by the exchange of energy between subatomic particles.[5]

According to the Big Bang theory, in the first tiny fractions of a second that the Big Bang occurred, there were no particles of matter, only "virtual particles,"[6] which appeared fleetingly, to exchange energy with other quantum particles, combining and destroying one another in the process, and causing arbitrary fluctuations of energy. This "subatomic tango,"[7] as Lynne McTaggart calls it in her book *The Field: The Quest for the Secret Force of the Universe*,[8] still takes place today; these particles fizz in and out of existence in a vacuum. Quantum mechanics has shown that that *vacuum* is not nothingness, as so many of us assume, but instead a flurry of quantum activity. This ground state is a system at the temperature of zero, called zero-point energy, which is the lowest possible energy state, when matter has been removed and nothing is supposedly left to create motion.[9]

"The zero-point energy in any one particular transaction in an electromagnetic field is unimaginably tiny—half a photon's worth," explains McTaggart. "But if you add up all the particles in the universe constantly popping in and out of being, you come up with a vast, inexhaustible energy source—equal to or greater than the energy density in an atomic nucleus—all sitting there unobtrusively in the background of empty space around us, like one [all-pervasive], supercharged backdrop."[10] This supercharged backdrop is the zero point field, or as it's sometimes referred to, the field of fields. These quantum calculations demonstrate that we live amidst a vast and constant sea of energy. This sea of energy, as the physicist Hal Puthoff illustrated in 1990,[11] is in dynamic relationship with all of the subatomic particles of the universe. The movement of each drives the other forward. This interaction "constitutes an underlying, stable . . . vacuum state," declared Puthoff, "in which further ZPF interaction simply reproduces the existing state on a dynamic-equilibrium basis."[12] The ZPF, in other words, is constantly renewing, and is constantly renewed by, the quantum movement of the universe. This also suggests that the universe—and all matter within it—is connected by the waves of the zero point field, and the boundless reservoir of energy that underlies it.

Which, to me, sounds a lot like the Tao.

In energy medicine, it is believed that there is a field that encompasses the body as a whole. The Chinese call this qi. It is this field—also sometimes referred to as the etheric field—that a skilled energy worker can influence in order to improve a patient's health. Though there isn't conclusive evidence of this energy field, the same is true of the now scientifically accepted notion of a gravitational field; scientists infer that the gravitational field exists because it offers a systematic, and reasonable, explanation for the way in which objects exist in space.

And yet the energy field of the body does have scientific relevance. In 1935, Harold S. Burr, a professor of anatomy at Yale University School of Medicine, conducted a series of experiments on animals—such as salamanders and chicks[13]—using a specially adapted voltmeter, designed to read very small voltages in order to detect the electric potential of the body. He concluded that all living systems had bioelectric fields. His own name for this was the L-field, which stood for "field of life."[14] Burr believed not only that life exhibited electromagnetic properties but that these comprised the "organizing principle"[15] that kept our bodies from falling into chaos. Our individual electromagnetic fields maintain a pattern that provides the "wholeness, organization and continuity" of all our bodily systems.[16]

In 1939, at around the same time that Burr was conducting his research, Semyon Kirlian, an electrician in the Soviet city of Krasnodar, stumbled across what he came to believe was photographic evidence of the human energy field.[17] While making an electrical repair at a medical research institute, he observed patients being treated with electrotherapy; he noticed that tiny flashes of light were visible between the electrodes and skin of the patients during their treatment. Intrigued as to what this could mean, Kirlian decided to try to capture it on his own at home. He placed photographic paper between electrodes and the skin of his hand and took an image. When he developed the photograph, he discovered that a luminescent glow surrounded his hand and fingers.

Kirlian learned that there was a scientific phrase for what he thought he had picked up on film: corona discharge. "*Corona*," from the ancient Greek, means a garland or wreath; it is the aura of plasma that rings the sun and other stars. But "corona discharge" is a term used in physics to describe the electrical glow on or around a charged conductor.[18] Kirlian believed he had captured the corona discharge coming off of his hand. As he adapted this method, placing an object between a metal plate and a piece of photographic paper while applying a high-voltage current to the metal plate—a process that has since come to be known as Kirlian photography—he discovered that inanimate objects, such as a coin, gave off a different coronal discharge; it was more of a uniform glow.[19] But living things—such as himself or a plant—created vivid, multicolored discharges, sending off flares of turquoise and maroon and purple. These were, Kirlian concluded, photographic stills of the vibrating energy field that surrounds all living things.

In an experiment that became one of the more famous of Kirlian's investigations, he took a picture of a fresh leaf—displaying its brightly colored "aura"—and then cut it in half and took a second photograph. In this photograph, again there was an aura, but instead of it lighting up around the remaining half of the leaf only, it continued to glow around the entire shape of it, in spite of the fact that half of it was now missing. This became known as the phantom leaf effect[20]—and has since been replicated and referred to reliably by practitioners of alternative medicine as proof of an energy field that surrounds the body.

This theory has also since been denounced by the scientific world.[21] The counterexplanation is that the high-voltage frequency applied to the metal plate rips the electrons off of atoms, causing the air around the photographed object to become ionized. If that air contains any water, this will cause a glowing silhouette around the object. The more water, the stronger the silhouette. The cause of the phantom leaf effect, then, was residual moisture left where half of the leaf had been torn away. Soon after, however, a researcher at California State University expanded on Kirlian's leaf experiment by photographing the missing part of the leaf through a clear Lucite block, which moisture could not pass through.[22] And the vibrant silhouette of the entire leaf still appeared in the image. As with much of science, there isn't a conclusive answer here, only evidence that can offer us different perspectives for understanding what we can't yet know for certain.

And yet, other scientific observations suggest that Kirlian may have been onto something. In fact, some of Harold Burr's research powerfully complements Kirlian's work. Many of Burr's experiments were performed on salamanders, useful in the lab in large part because they are observable from the egg stage through to adulthood, allowing for changes in form to be observed and noted with precision. Using his voltmeter, Burr discovered that salamander eggs have an electrical energy field nearly identical to the shape of the animal itself.[23] Given this, Burr theorized that the electrical energy field axis—the central line around which this energy revolves—would align with the nervous system of an adult salamander. To explore this, he injected droplets of dark, indelible ink into the energy field axis in a series of salamander eggs. In each case, he found that the ink became incorporated into the brain and spinal cord of the developing salamander. This was a radical and provocative finding: Did this mean salamanders possess their adult energetic blueprint at birth? It was as if the salamander held, in embryo, the energetic outline of its future self.

There is also evidence that the reverse could be true (along the lines of Kirlian's leaf study): an electrical field remains *after* limbs have been lost. Robert O. Becker, an orthopedic surgeon, published research throughout the 1940s and 1950s, primarily in the *Journal of Bone and Joint Surgery*, that illustrated a "current of injury," meaning an electric current from the central part of the body to an injured nerve or muscle, in animals. The injured tissue registered a negative voltage as compared to the rest of the body.[24]

Becker, too, used salamanders in his studies because they are one of the few animals that can regenerate limbs. Yes, an adult salamander whose leg is removed will, over the course of a few weeks, grow a brand-new one where there was once just a stump! Becker also examined frogs, by comparison, in order to study an animal not capable of this kind of regrowth. When Becker amputated both animals' limbs, he found that they generated the same current of injury, a positive voltage. But, soon after, he found that the salamander developed a change of charge at its stump: switching from a positive to a negative polarity before declining—indicating an energetic potential—and then, once the regeneration of the limb was complete, climbing back to zero. The frog's voltage, meanwhile, went to zero when the leg was amputated and remained there as the stump scarred over.[25]

Before I'd even come across these studies, I had a patient in hospice who once told me he was feeling pain in a leg he no longer had. I asked him to lie down and, acting on instinct, began to treat his missing leg. I simply placed the needles on the bed, where his acupuncture points would have been, along what is called the "gallbladder channel," which stretches the length of the leg down to the foot. After about ten minutes, he remarked that he thought the pain was decreasing. "It is?" I asked, quietly incredulous. By the end of the treatment, after an hour or so, he described the pain as having gone from an eight (out of ten) to a three. At the time, though startled my impromptu plan had worked, I explained it to myself as the placebo effect. He'd believed the acupuncture would help him, I thought, and so it had. But I've since come to believe that my acupuncture needles made small electrical interventions in a part of his body that was no longer there. In other words, it was possible to affect the field—and move the energy—enveloping his missing leg.

The electromagnetic force, as understood in conventional biomedicine, governs the fleeting interactions between molecules; bioelectromagnetics, however, calls upon electromagnetic, electric, and magnetic fields to explain an all-encompassing field used to regulate life functions. Energy medicine takes the understanding of the electromagnetic fields one step further, proposing that an energetic exchange between practitioner and patient can have a healing outcome.

As I became more conscious of something running through me in my early days of practicing acupuncture, my patients began to sense it too. Many described feeling a sensation of heat and movement. I was treating everything from chronic pain to allergies as well as, increasingly, women with fertility issues—all with impressive results. In particular, as I saw these women's hormones come into balance, their uterine linings thicken appropriately, and menstrual cycles regulate, I wondered if I was offering their bodies information that allowed their reproductive systems to reorganize.

It also occurred to me that my own body might be affected in this process. Around this time, I'd put on a good deal of weight (though my eating habits hadn't changed), and I also dealt with spontaneous and aggressive bouts of an irregular heartbeat called tachycardia. Every few months, I would be in the middle of a normal day, treating patients in my clinic, when suddenly instead of feeling the energy flow through me as usual, I would feel as if I were about to have a heart attack.

When my tachycardia was diagnosed, I also discovered that I have a genetic disorder called Wolff-Parkinson-White Syndrome, which means I was born with an extra row of the cells that conduct electrical activity in the heart. (I sometimes joke that this gives me extra heart qi.) It's a congenital condition, but I had no symptoms until I started channeling energy while practicing acupuncture. I could often control the tachycardia on my own—by rubbing the carotid artery in my neck and putting ice on my face, both well-established methods for reducing heart rate taught to me by my former paramedic husband. Still, on a couple of occasions the episodes were severe enough that I had to be rushed to the emergency room. There, the doctors administered adenosine intravenously, causing what is known as asystole—or cardiac arrest—for a few seconds. Ultimately, this allows the heart to re-establish a normal rhythm. Along the way, however, it also incites excruciating chest pain, not to mention the morbid realization that this may be the end.

Perhaps I was having these tachycardia incidents because I was overworked, but I couldn't shake the instinct that my heart was actually having trouble adjusting to what felt like I was picking up different frequencies from the fields surrounding me. There are, in fact, fields that emanate from *within* us. Our brains and hearts, for example, each have their own measurable electromagnetic fields. Medical doctors track the vibrating field of the brain with an electroencephalogram, or EEG. Our brain cells also communicate using electrical impulses, which are always active, even when we sleep; these movements show up as the wavy lines on an EEG reading, a measurement of frequency.

The heart, however, projects the largest electromagnetic field in the body. This can be measured using an electrocardiogram, also called an ECG or EKG. The heart's field is so impressive, in fact, that modern medical equipment can now measure its frequency from up to fifteen feet away.[26]

Through their pulsating fields, these two organs—the heart and the brain—are always communicating. Medical doctors carefully track the energy fields of the heart and the brain individually, but pay less attention to the ways the two affect each other electromagnetically. There are, however, researchers—such as Dr. Gary Schwartz, a professor of psychiatry and medicine at the University of Arizona, and a group called the HeartMath Institute,[27] founded by both scientists and energy healers—who have pioneered a movement to investigate this connection.

Schwartz and his colleagues Drs. Linda Russek and Linda Song—conducting experiments that simultaneously tracked the EEG and EKG readings of participants—found that when participants were asked to concentrate on their heartbeats there was not only an increased sensing of the heart signal in their brain waves generally but also a heightened registration of the P-wave, which is the first part of the heartbeat, when blood is pumped to the ventricles, and is difficult to feel physiologically.[28] This offers evidence that, as Schwartz writes, "when we focus our attention on our hearts, our brains amplify the electrical fields coming from our hearts even during those moments—the P-wave periods—when sensations from the heart have yet to reach our brains."[29] Stated another way, the brain has an implicit perception of the heart that bypasses the known communication pathways in the body. I wondered if this inherent communication between the brain and the heart held a clue as to the accommodations my body was making when energy flowed through me.

The Chinese philosopher Lao Tzu once said, "When the student is ready, the teacher will appear," and I have found this to be true in my life. In this case, my teacher appeared in the form of a clinical and sports psychologist named Leah Lagos.* She reached out to me after I'd treated one of her patients, an actress who was struggling with stage fright. She told me she had seen a "measurable change"[30] in her patient's condition and invited me to come to her office to discuss my work. My curiosity was piqued. Among other things, I was interested to find out what exactly she was measuring, so we arranged a meeting.

* http://www.drleahlagos.com/.

Dr. Lagos is a specialist in heart rate variability (HRV) biofeed-back,[31] which she uses to help patients improve cardiac health as well as to teach techniques for dealing with anxiety. A large number of her clients are professional athletes, CEOs, and actors—those who execute the emotional equivalent of a high-wire act every time they go out in front of an audience; they must be in control of their thoughts and emotions in order to do their jobs.

We tend to think of a healthy heartbeat as being regular, but in reality the heart varies the time between beats as it adapts to changing circumstances. Lagos identifies these variations, using an EKG machine, in order to document when a person is breathing at a rate that produces optimum heart rate variability: "When you inhale, your heart rate goes up, and when you exhale, your heart rate goes down," she says. "You want these oscillations to be as big as possible, but you also want them to be orderly. When you're stressed, frustrated, upset, your heart rate becomes erratic. When you are relaxed, you have this beautiful, ocean-like wave. Since your heart is a muscle, this movement can be acquired."[32] Her protocol, which allows her patients, as she puts it, "to gain the ability to control their physiology and psychology through their heart rhythms,"[33] is a ten-week program—which includes meeting in her office once a week and doing breathing exercises twice a day. Lagos believes that the heart is at the center of emotional control and has been overlooked by an insistent focus on the brain. (She also envisions a future in which people will see their *psychophysiologists* weekly instead of their psychotherapists.)

Ultimately, Lagos aims to alter the body's autonomic nervous system response to stress. The autonomic nervous system has two primary reactions: sympathetic and parasympathetic.

When you're scurrying across a busy intersection and the light changes, setting a number of cars in motion, the body goes into fight-or-flight mode, which is also known as the sympathetic response. This is a valuable response: it amps you up and urges you to sprint to the sidewalk before the cars reach you. But once you've reached the sidewalk, if you don't have a strong parasympathetic response to bring you back into balance, you remain in that survival state for longer than is necessary. For those who are chronically stressed, this can last for hours and sometimes even days. Lagos's regimen helps her patients to bolster the parasympathetic response—encouraging more heart rate variability and a lower heart rate—in order to interrupt the sympathetic reaction sooner.

"Think of a tennis player getting ready for the US Open: they're not thinking about which muscles to exercise—that's what muscle memory is, and it's the same thing with the heart," Lagos explains. "Enough repetitions at a specific frequency, the heart embraces the pattern and functionally kicks into it on its own at stressful moments. It changes your reactivity and response to stress."[34]

Lagos studies her patients' heart frequencies by measuring electrical activity of the heart with an EKG as they breathe at a specific pace. When breathing rate and heart rate coincide, maximizing heart rate oscillations, a patient has reached what she considers an ideal state: they are in resonance. "When you are breathing at your resonant frequency, you're strengthening the parasympathetic influence to come in and break that fight-or-flight tendency," says Lagos, "and bring you back to homeostasis."[35] During resonance, the rhythms of the heart create calming signals that reverberate throughout the entire autonomic nervous system.

Resonance is an important concept in physics too. Defined broadly, it is when one object vibrates at the same natural frequency of a second object, thereby increasing the amplitude and forcing the second object into vibrational motion. It is the reason the wineglass shatters when the opera singer hits an extraordinarily high note. (The word "resonance" comes from the Latin term meaning "echo" or "resound.") When the singer's voice reaches a certain earsplitting pitch—one that matches the resonant frequency of the glass—the resulting vibration breaks it. In Lagos's office, however, coming into a state of resonance is the opposite of shattering: it is in fact when a person is operating at the height of her powers.

When Lagos had seen the actress, our mutual patient, after I had given her an acupuncture treatment with energy work, she'd noticed that she'd gone into resonance much more easily than before, as measured by her biofeedback instruments. She wanted to know what I had done that had made a difference. I explained to her what acupuncture points I'd treated and also acknowledged that I'd been feeling an energy come through me for some time while practicing acupuncture. We decided to hook me up to the biofeedback equipment to see if we might glean any information. When Lagos attached the EKG nodes, I instinctively went into the state I enter when I am healing—and, within fifteen seconds, I was in resonance. Apparently, I'd naturally, and blindly, stumbled into training myself to do this as I practiced acupuncture. Lagos theorized that I'd come to this naturally because my increased heart rate variability offered me a greater flexibility to open to and transfer energy to my patients.

Intrigued by this result, Lagos invited me back for an additional assessment—a concomitant EEG of my brain and an EKG of my heart. Again, almost immediately, my brain and heart went into resonance with each other. These experiments in Lagos's office helped me to understand that what I was feeling during healing sessions was the result of a measurable change in my breath, heartbeat, and brain waves. This was a significant finding, suggesting that my entire autonomic nervous system was acclimating during my healing sessions. The most obvious way to do this is through the vagus nerve, which links the heart and the brain and helps the parasympathetic nervous system restore order in the heart and respiratory system as well as the digestive system after a stressful event.

Lagos agreed that my tachycardia might have been the result of my unconsciously practicing this technique in my sessions. While it put me into resonance, it may also have occasionally affected my vagus nerve, which would create a rapid heartbeat. And, because of my Wolff-Parkinson-White Syndrome, this sometimes became out of control. The balance between the parasympathetic and sympathetic systems is a delicate dance for anyone. Most of the time, I was able to pull it off, but every once in a while, as energy came through me, I believe my body wasn't able to adapt appropriately. I might have also found a way to modulate my autonomic nervous system in order to align with

my patients, syncing to their frequencies and establishing a resonance with them.

At least that was my instinct, and although it may sound improbable, it's not an entirely unscientific hypothesis. Dr. Gary
Schwartz also had a feeling that, given the heart's powerful electromagnetic field, we might be able to pick up signals from others.
Schwartz has enough humor—and humility—to suggest some
might find this to be "the new age musing of an aging researcher,"[36]
but he also has the integrity of his scientific background, urging
him to seek evidence-based confirmation of his beliefs.

As such, he analyzed the EKG and EEG readings of a researcher, Dr. Russek, and twenty male participants. All of these
men had taken part in a study forty years prior, when they were
students at Harvard. In that initial experiment, they were asked
to rate their mother and fathers on a numerical scale, in six positive traits: loving, just, fair, clever, hardworking, and strong.

Schwartz found that "if the subjects perceived their parents as
loving when they were in college, they made an energetic connection with the interviewer that meant they registered the presence of the interviewer's heart waves in their brain waves when
they were mature adults."[37] On the other hand, the brain waves
of participants who'd rated their parents with low scores in the
"loving" category linked with the interviewer's heart waves in
weaker and more delayed ways. These results were replicated
when the HeartMath Institute performed the experiment again
independently.[38]

This research signifies a profound concept: that one person's
heart waves, issuing from their heart's electromagnetic field,
can detect—and affect—another person's brain waves, and vice

versa. I believe that this may also be happening when I perform treatments in my clinic: just as Dr. Lagos found that I went into internal resonance when I was in clinic, this research suggests that I may also go into resonance with my patients, meaning our heart waves and brain waves synchronize temporarily during the course of a healing treatment.

Further evidence of this can be found in research showing that changes purposefully induced in one person's brain can naturally effect a similar change in another person's brain. Specifically, in a study reported in *Science* in 1965, two researchers looked at the EEG results of fifteen pairs of identical twins who were sitting in separate rooms. In two of these pairs, when alpha rhythms, the electrical oscillations in the brain that occur when a person is awake and relaxed, were deliberately induced in one identical twin by researchers, they spontaneously and simultaneously occurred in the other.[39]

More recently, in 2010, three researchers—Dr. Luke Hendricks, Dr. William Bengston, and Dr. Jay Gunkelman—studied a distance healer working with patients placed in rooms thirty-five feet away, simultaneously tracking the electrical signals of their brains through EEGs.[40] They found that the healer possessed an electromagnetic standing wave of around 7.81 Hz, which was stronger and more frequent than that of the patients. After a while, however, the patients' wave frequencies appeared to reset and synchronize to the same as that of the healer. In other words, resonance occurred between the healer and patient, even when separated. And the bond between the healer and the patient created a measurably more powerful resonance than either individual was capable of alone.

Bengston did a follow-up study at the University of Connecticut, which he later replicated at Thomas Jefferson University's Sidney Kimmel Medical College, in which he, himself, practiced a meditative exercise for healing while hooked up to an EEG.[41] At the same time, another person was wired to a separate EEG machine. While Bengston was engaging in the meditative exercise, a measurable difference occurred in the second person's brain that matched that of Bengston's EEG reading. When Bengston stopped the mental exercise, this synchronization of brain waves stopped as well.

These experiments suggest that the energy fields of our hearts and brains can—and do—reach others. We are, in essence, in quiet collaboration with one another.

There is another body of scientific research that indicates that we may all be connected in an essential but imperceptible way. The Princeton Engineering Anomalies Research (PEAR) program was a lab under the aegis of Princeton University's School of Engineering and Applied Science that dedicated nearly three decades to the research of human consciousness and its effect—in particular, whether collective consciousness has the power to alter the course of events. The late Robert Jahn, a physicist who was then the dean of the engineering school at Princeton, founded PEAR in 1979 after an undergraduate requested that he oversee her study of the impact of human intention on a mechanical device—in this case, a small, boxlike machine called a random event generator (REG), designed to produce a stream of unpredictable digital bits, translated to ones or zeros on a computer that serves as a database.[42] Simply put, this device is like an electronic coin toss with a fifty-fifty chance of producing a one or a zero.

Jahn was primarily interested in the REG itself—he thought examining its design would be a good independent study for this student—but as his student's work progressed, he became increasingly drawn in by her data and results. Over the ensuing decades, with Brenda Dunne—a developmental psychologist who became PEAR's laboratory manager—working by his side, Jahn and his staff conducted thousands of experiments. Devising their own, more sophisticated version of the machine, they studied the REG in a variety of circumstances and settings, aiming to determine whether humans could make a difference on the outpouring of numbers.

And they did. The difference, on average, is the equivalent to someone being able to alter the outcome of a coin toss every two to three flips per ten thousand.[43] It's a small but, statistically speaking, significant number. "The phenomena are real," Dunne says. "They are not chance fluctuations. There is a subtle ordering process that is influencing these otherwise random events."[44] Jahn and his staff conducted thousands of experiments with the REG over the twenty-eight-year span that the lab was in operation: in almost every one, the statistical difference was slightly higher than it would have been in the case of a purely random set of numbers.[45]

The PEAR lab came to believe that these anomalies were strongly associated with two factors: if there was an intention or need on behalf of the person operating the machine, and if there was a strong feeling of resonance—meaning, in this context, that the frequencies of two electromagnetic fields (either between two people or between a person and the machine) aligned.*

The PEAR lab experiments have also explored the effects on the REG when a single person and when a couple—romantically involved and not—were paired with the machine, offering prestated intentions beforehand. The results showed that in either scenario, human electromagnetic fields could affect those of the machine; interestingly, two people create a stronger effect than one, and a couple with an emotional attachment produces the most notable results. As Jahn once said, "If you get your mind in resonance with the processor, it will show a preference for following your desire."[46]

The PEAR lab studied resonance within groups as well. "We developed a little portable REG that we could take out into the field," Dunne explains, "and we would take it to different environments where there was likely to be a strong collective resonance."[47] The settings ranged from a conference on humor to musical concerts to meditation groups—events that were considered "charismatic." Again, the numbers showed a slight but significant pattern; they were more organized than the purely random numbers offered by the control group. By contrast, more subdued events, such as academic conferences and business meetings, showed less deviation.

The PEAR lab ended its investigations in 2007. "We have accomplished what we originally set out to do . . . namely to de-

---

* The relationship between the mind and a machine is becoming increasingly more critical. Companies like Cyberkinetics have, for the last twenty years, been developing the technology to create brain-computer interfaces (BMIs), which are chips that can be inserted into the brain to allow a person to control electronic devices with the mind.

termine whether these effects are real and to identify their major correlates," Jahn and Dunne said in a joint statement. "It is time for the next generation of scholars to take over."

Since then, Roger Nelson, an experimental psychologist with a background in physics and statistical methods, who was also the operations coordinator at PEAR, created the Global Consciousness Project (GCP).[48] This is an international project that expands upon the work of PEAR, though it functions independently of it. The group has installed a network of REGs around the world—from France to New Zealand to Kenya to New York—all of which send data continuously to a server in Princeton, New Jersey. These machines are a bit like electrodes, as Nelson describes it, "taking the EEG of the planet."[49] Ultimately, the GCP seeks to measure the effects of the global collective consciousness.

To do so, researchers examine the data from the machines at the time of riveting world events, ranging in variety from New Year's Eve to the 2010 earthquake in Haiti to Donald Trump's 2016 inauguration.[50] "We are looking at times when groups of people became resonant with each other," Nelson explains. "We identify an occurrence that we think represents a moment in time when people really came together and shared emotions in a profound way"[51]—and then create a statistical analysis of the information streaming from the machines during that time.

Specifically, they determine the mean output from the various REGs scattered about the world, determining whether the numbers adhere to a baseline, or if they increase or decrease. The formal measure looks at pair-wise correlations. They compare the data from the New York REG with every other machine in the network, for example—to see if there is any correlation within pairs.

Statistically, there shouldn't be a correlation at all beyond a very small variation above or below zero. But the GCP has found that many of these events have incurred parallels between information coming from different machines.[52]

On New Year's Eve, for example, they have discovered the data, if mapped, reliably creates a V-shaped curve, with midnight represented by the bottom point of the V.[53] That is, the machines tend to correlate during the worldwide rise in excitement leading up to midnight and then again as the tension dissipates just after midnight.

"Nobody has a fully adequate theory for why this happens," Nelson acknowledges. "But I think we each have our individual consciousness . . . We imagine it is in our heads, maybe in the brain—but the experience of thousands of years and recent scientific empirical evidence indicates that the mind extends out into the world. Consciousness is not a confined unity or entity stuck inside the skin and bone; it is much more expansive."[54]

The GCP also analyzes their findings by categories, breaking the events down by size and whether the event elicited positive or negative emotions. Compassion, Nelson notes, seems to be one of the strongest determinants for correlation. "It is an emotion that does connect us—and we find events that evoke compassion yield larger data deviations,"[55] he explains. "But fear is also quite strong. I wish I could say fear doesn't do anything but it, too, causes a kind of interconnection."

Sometimes the two emotions are intertwined, as with 9/11. The GCP found their numbers showed a sharp variation during this crisis, although the trend started about four or five hours *before* the first plane hit and lasted for three days afterward.

Though Nelson makes clear that it is not a scientific conclusion, he interprets this early statistical deviation as a collective premonition and the sustained shift afterward as a reflection of the world's continuing intense emotions. Critics, however, point to this as an example of the unreliability of the results and a bias toward retrofitting them with an explanation. Whatever the case may be, the statistical deviations during the formal database of five hundred specified world events are calculated by the GCP to be one-in-a-trillion odds that they could happen only by chance.

"We're a little like neurons. There are one hundred billion neurons in the human brain. When they do their job, the result is an incredibly unexpected new thing we experience as consciousness and reflection and emotion," Nelson says. "Soon there will be ten billion people in the world; we are designed to be interconnected. And there is a potential awakening for us, to reach a more unified field of consciousness, to create a layer of intelligence for the earth. I think it's important that we acknowledge that we are interconnected in some way, to accept that and learn from it."[56]

Though it's not yet possible to wholly explain the effects of energy medicine through the lens of science—the healing relationship contains intangible elements that will always remain mysterious—it is clear to me that the practice obeys the laws of physics in significant ways. Practically speaking, we are all connected through our electromagnetic fields, be it of our whole bodies or those of our brains or our hearts, but I believe—as the work of Dr. Gary Schwartz, the HeartMath Institute, and the PEAR lab also suggest—that we are able to affect one another with our energy fields. We are, in this way, creating a communal movement that, as the Global Consciousness Project is seeking to measure, ebbs and flows on a tide of collective emotion. Like Einstein's "spooky actions at a distance," we are connected in ways that can be glimpsed, and even partially explained, through science. The mystery remains largely in the universal energy field—what Chinese philosophy calls the Tao and quantum physics calls the zero point field—which I believe is intelligent. This larger energy field is interacting with us at all times; we are in a kind of conversation with it. It has a degree of governance over our lives, but we can also influence it with our thoughts and actions. Recent scientific research is offering a glimpse of a phenomenon religious people have taken on faith, that there is an unseen force that we experience, and can be altered by, whether we are conscious of it or not.

YOU THE HEALER

Resonant Breathing

Research suggests that healers adapt their physiology in order to heal. In my case, as Dr. Lagos discovered, the frequencies of my brain and heart begin to resonate. Further research has shown that patients then mirror the healer and as their frequencies align a resonant bond is created. This bond seems to be the optimal connection for the transfer of energetic information. The first stage of this process is to practice a breathing technique that encourages internal resonance. Here is the exercise Dr. Lagos gives her patients. It's simple but effective.

The optimal breathing rate to create the most heart rate variability is five breaths per minute. This means that each inhale and exhale lasts six seconds.

Practice breathing in gently for a count of six and then breathing out smoothly, also for a count of six. Don't force it. The goal here is to balance your sympathetic nervous system—the one responsible for your fight-or-flight response—with your parasympathetic nervous system, which slows your heart rate down. For the same reason, I recommend that you don't count aloud or use a visual cue (such as an app) to keep track of your breaths, as it could mildly activate your sympathetic nervous system.

3

WHAT'S GOD GOT
TO DO WITH IT?

My mother tried to take her own life once. This was thirty years before she actually died, during one of the blackest periods of her depression; she took an overdose of pills after a series of arguments with my grandmother. I was at home—though too young to understand what was happening—when my father found her unconscious in the bath and called an ambulance so she could be rushed to the hospital.

My mother later said that while she was on the gurney in the hospital, with the doctors working to revive her, she left her body. She felt drawn out of herself, pulled toward a light, and she could see herself below with the doctors gathered around her. In the presence of that light, she told me, she felt the safest she'd ever felt. And she heard voices. They told her she should go back, that she had two small children who needed her, but they also said this had to be her choice. She had to *choose* to go back to her life.

She struggled with the choice of leaving such unmitigated comfort and protection to return to the sharp-edged pain of her life, but in the end, she did decide to come back to us, her children. And when she did, she felt suddenly flung back into her body. She opened her eyes to see the doctors, gathered above her now, having just resuscitated her.

My mother told me this story when I was still a child, only ten years old. I later recognized, after my work in the hospice, that she'd had a classic near-death experience. Back when my mother had this experience—before people spoke openly of such incidents and long before the Internet became our ubiquitous source of information—my mother had no idea that many other people had experienced a similar phenomenon. But I regularly heard similar stories from my patients in the days before they died. Some, like my mother, saw a numinous light and felt a similar sense of consoling tranquility, while others encountered a more fully realized vision of heaven or dead family members. One of my patients was a seven-year-old boy—not all hospices take pediatric cases, but ours did—with a rare form of bone cancer. He told his mother in the midst of his dying that he could see his granny, his mother's mother, who'd passed away years before. "You should go to her," his mother said, generously guiding him toward the very place she did not want him to go.

There are a handful of explanations that scientists offer to explain what happens in a near-death experience (NDE)—a shortage of oxygen can cause hallucinations; a stressed brain can produce endorphins that might create a sense of peace; a damaged part of the brain called the temporoparietal junction, which contributes to our overall perception of our bodies, could trigger a sense of being outside of the body. And yet none of these theories offers definitive evidence that a near-death experience is simply the elaborate fantasy of an addled brain—nor do they explain why the stories are all so alike. Some NDE researchers are doctors and neuroscientists who, having experienced such an incident themselves, suggest that these occurrences reveal our essential selves, something within us that isn't inextricably bound up in our neural circuitry.[1]

I believe that this departing piece of us is our energetic aspect, also called the spirit or soul. The similarity of NDE accounts suggests to me that when our energy is leaving our bodies, we experience a fleeting connection with the universal energy field. I most often call this field "source," because it is just that—a starting point, a fount, the origin—but others call it God or Yahweh or Allah or Brahma or, for those with less of an inclination toward the mystic, the zero point field. In Chinese philosophy, it is, as we've discussed, referred to as the Tao, which translates roughly to "the way." Truly, *it* can be called anything—and nothing at all. There is an expression in Chinese philosophy that beautifully captures what I mean: "The Tao that can be spoken of is not the eternal Tao."[2]

As my acupuncture business grew, I felt an increasing belief in my practice *and* an increasing sense of pressure. I had arrived in New York with a rosy enthusiasm intact: I thought I would do good things, help people to heal, and the world would line up to support me. In truth, of course, it wasn't that straightforward.

Though my abilities were expanding, I hadn't yet learned how to manage them responsibly. I couldn't bring myself to turn away a single patient, so I was booking sessions back-to-back, offering more of myself than I could afford to give; I was depleted and overwhelmed. I was also ill-equipped to run the business side of my acupuncture practice. I spent so much time building a trust and affinity with patients—creating an atmosphere for healing in clinic—it was difficult for me to shift roles outside of that to make practical decisions. This soon took its toll. Most painfully, a colleague with whom I'd been working on a project for more than a year passed our work off as his own, and started a competing venture. I've since accepted that in business, as in life, I will inevitably interact with someone who has the potential to be a bit of a wild card, but, at that time, I felt completely blindsided.

I recalled a book called *Conversations with God*[3] a friend had once left behind in my home. I'd picked it up and skimmed the first page—and found I couldn't put it down. The author, despite using the word "God," offered nondenominational, nonjudgmental guidance that spoke to me in the most clear and startling way and, I later realized, put words to some of the most powerful experiences in my energy work.

I reached out to Neale Donald Walsch, the author of that book, under the auspices of a work project having to do with the variety of ways we define God. When we finally connected, however, we talked instead about how drained I felt and the anxiety I had about the future. In the middle of our conversation, perhaps sensing that I was not at a point where I would be embarking on a new project of any kind, Neale asked me point-blank, "Do you need a mentor?"

And we began our enlightening friendship.

. . .

In the early 1990s, Neale was entering his fifties when he went through a crucible of sorts: his house caught on fire, destroying all of his belongings; his marriage fell apart; and he was in a serious car accident that left him with a broken neck. Once he'd recovered physically and was able to take a look around, he saw his life had been torn asunder. He was alone, homeless, and unemployed. He began living in a tent just outside of Ashland, Oregon. Eventually he scraped together enough money to rent a small cottage, and while there in the spring of 1992, Neale picked up a legal pad and began to write an angry letter to God, lamenting his bad luck.

And God answered.

"To my surprise, as I scribbled out the last of my bitter, unanswerable questions and prepared to toss my pen aside, my hand remained poised over the paper, as if held there by some invisible force,"[4] Neale wrote in what would become *Conversations with God*, the first book in a three-part series that has since been translated into thirty-seven languages. ". . . I had no idea what I was about to write, but an idea seemed to be coming, so I decided to flow with it."[5]

What followed was a surprising, fresh, searching conversation—with Neale asking the difficult questions and someone, *something*, that he experienced as God, offering him answers that he wrote down, exactly (as he later described it) as a person taking dictation. The tone of this God is not threatening or punishing or abstract, but humane and accessible.

I did once ask Neale, now in his seventies with a kind of celestial handsomeness, why he thought his communicator, this voice that had spoken to him, chose to call itself God, a name that makes some people, including me, flinch a little. My resistance is rooted in the Methodist church of my childhood, where my grandmother was a lay preacher; she, along with our church community, often used God as a representation of, and justification for, their judgments, creating a punitive sense of faith. I understood this even as a girl in England, and, as an adult, I've come to realize religion, in general, can be limiting. In some cases, as with the Methodist church of my childhood, this is due to the dogma attached to the story of their faith; other times, it is because religion often anthropomorphizes what I see as an energy that is broader and more adaptive in relation to us. Though, on the whole, I think we're all perceiving the same thing: there is an intelligent force that is overseeing us in some way. In my view, this force, or energy field—or source—is a bit more unpredictable because it also responds to what we are putting out with our own energy fields, individually and collectively.

To this end, Neale responded to my question by saying that we don't need to stop using the word "God," but rather consider what the true meaning of the word is. "Where *is* God in all of this?" he asked. "This is the central question facing humanity. Is there something we do not fully understand here, the understanding of which would change everything?"[6]

I told Neale how angry I was—how absurdly, unshakably angry— about the man who'd claimed my work as his own, stealing my clients and leaving my business in precarious financial standing. I'd been lying awake night after night, I told him, grinding my teeth, and thinking of how this man—someone to whom I'd generously offered my time and energy and creativity—had taken so much from me. Why did this happen? I asked Neale. What would his God say?

"If I was God," Neale said, "I'd suggest that you were being ungrateful. You have so much of what you want—your first book is a success, you've built a practice strong enough to survive these kinds of blows. What has he really taken from you? And what if this man came along so that you could learn to hone your ideas and develop an authentic way of communicating them to people?"[7] Basically, Neale urged me to be grateful for all that I already had but also, curiously, that this man had come into my life. "Gratitude is the most important piece, the most powerful tool in our tool chest that we've been given to get through the human experience," he said. "What you resist persists. But what you look at with gratitude ceases to have illusory form."[8]

What Neale was saying, I came to understand, was rooted in a deeper faith than the one I yet had. As God—or the Tao or source or whatever we'd like to call this divine support—explained to Neale, the process of constructing our lives "must include belief, or knowing. This is absolute faith. This is *beyond* hoping. . . . This place of knowing is a place of intense and incredible gratitude. It is a *thankfulness in advance*. And that, perhaps, is the biggest key to creation: to be grateful *before*, and for, the creation."[9]

Neale takes the notion of gratitude a step further, giving it a therapeutic twist. He says that it is not only important to remain grateful during the missteps and tragedies but that this act will actually move you forward. "When we stop resisting what we think is unwelcome in our lives, the very shifting of our interior energy begins to impact the exterior circumstance in a way that can be salvific," Neale told me. "It can turn things around."

And, just like that, I dropped this resentment that had haunted me for a year. I poured myself a glass of wine, raised it to the man who had conned me, and said, "Thank you." And I meant it. I finally understood that, although the path had been bumpy, everything was as it should be. It was deceptively simple advice in that it offered such profound effects. This man hadn't taken anything essential from me, after all. This cleared the path for me to see that I *was* thoroughly grateful for the life I was already leading. Every so often I would hear of a new way he'd used my work to promote his business venture and, while each betrayal would once again take my breath away, I was always able to move past my anger into gratitude.

In addition to gratitude, belief is also impactful. "Belief attracts to us what we firmly expect it to," Neale explained. This held true with my letting go. Once I believed this man wasn't able to diminish me, then, well, he was no longer able to diminish me. I'd been offering him the power to do so, and now I was taking it back. But, in a deeper sense, *belief,* to me, meant surrendering to the mystery of the energy I felt come through me in clinic—which, I have come to understand, I draw from source. I needed to accept, I realized, that this was a positive force that I did not have to fear or try to control.

Gratitude and belief are incompatible with any kind of yearning because, within that, there is an original, or hidden, thought—what Neale (and Neale's God) would call a Sponsoring Thought. This original thought—that you are, say, a person who cannot get what you want or is beset by tragedy—actually becomes the reality. This may sound like a riddle, but the basic tenet is that belief and gratitude should come from a place of *already* having as opposed to wanting more. If we are asking for something—*please stop letting bad things happen to me*—we're sending a message that we are in a state of deficiency and, therefore, that is what the universe will offer back. If we're in a state of gratitude, however, we're telling the universe that we already have what we want. Source is in conversation with us in this sense, contributing to the shape of our lives.

"You are a big creation machine, and you are turning out a new manifestation literally as fast as you can think,"[10] advises Neale's God. "Events, occurrences, happenings, conditions, circumstances—all are created out of consciousness. Individual consciousness is powerful enough. You can imagine what kind of creative energy is unleashed whenever two or more are gathered in My name. And *mass* consciousness? Why, *that* is so powerful it can create events and circumstances of worldwide import and planetary consequences. It would not be accurate to say—not in the way you mean it—that *you* are *choosing* these consequences. You are not choosing them anymore [*sic*] than I am choosing them. Like Me, you are observing them. And deciding Who You Are with regard to them."[11]

Initially, this is a matter of perception: if we alter our views in a more positive direction, we will likely feel better. But, once we truly change our emotions, we're also creating a new reality. (This, in essence, is what the Global Consciousness Project is tracking with its network of REGs around the world.) That is, we're all putting information out into the world that has the power to reshape not only our own lives but our collective circumstances as well. The key is that you must truly *feel* the shift toward gratitude—it cannot be a rote thought or tactic.

I was also interacting with source and effecting change, I realized, in just this way in my clinic. When I was with Andrew, my patient with prostate cancer, and I felt energy coming through me—that tingling sensation running through my spine—I recalled that if I thought to myself something like, *Please make Andrew healthy again*, or essentially asked for the power to heal him, the feeling would taper or vanish altogether. But if I was able to distract myself—and let go of my Sponsoring Thought, which communicated a sense of need—the energy flowed through me vigorously once more. This thought behind the thought, Neale taught and I now firmly believe, is the "raw energy that drives the engine of human experience."[12]

And, Neale explained, every Sponsoring Thought—really, every human thought and word and act—is based on fear or love. "Fear is the energy which contracts, closes down, draws in, hides, hoards, harms," he said. "Love is the energy which expands, opens up, sends out, reveals, shares, heals. You have free choice about which of these to select."

This was so clarifying to me—so straightforward yet also profoundly life-altering—I made a conscious choice before making every decision from then on, especially business decisions, as those were the ones about which I did not always have a clear instinct. I even began wearing a rubber band around my wrist so I could snap it whenever making a decision, to keep myself awake to the essential question: Love or fear?

. . .

And yet, despite these significant revelations, I kept coming up against the same challenge in my conversations with Neale. If there is a God, or source, one that wants to be responsive to us in positive ways, then why do such terrible things happen to good people? If I believe and I am grateful, and I choose love over fear, will that protect me? Had I chosen fear when I offered to work with the man who ultimately stole my work? Had my mother sided with fear when she struggled with depression? That Irishman who died in hospice had seemed as grateful as anyone I'd ever met—and yet he died at an age when most people are just starting to build their lives and families.

The specific answers were: Yes, you chose fear when you became fixated on the idea that this man had humiliated and deceived you. Your mother acted out of fear because she had perceived the world as hostile based on her difficult upbringing—which led to her depression. How do you know the Irishman did not have a peaceful death at home *because* he was grateful? Choosing love over fear does not protect us from the tumult of life, but it does influence our response to the hand we are dealt—and the way that the universe will shift its energy around us.

The broad answer was: We are one. We are all aspects of the same thing. We are here, each in our own physical incarnation, but with source uniting us. We experience a duality—yin and yang, matter and energy, good and bad—in order for source, and for us, to understand the full spectrum of the human experience. In Chinese philosophy, as I've mentioned, everything in the world has an opposite: Yin is the dark side of the mountain, whereas yang is the light. The two, yin and yang, are always in a state of dynamic balance in life and therefore always subtly—or sometimes not-so-subtly—changing. This could also be described as a shifting exchange between source and us and one another.

This, incidentally, is another way in which religion and energy healing part ways. Religion proposes a higher power, one that is separate from us, which creates, in Neale's words, "a separation theology: God is over there and we are over here, which creates a separation cosmology, which produces a separation psychology—I am separate from everybody else—which produces a separation sociology—entire societies believing they are separate—which inevitably produces a separation pathology observable in the human species from the beginning of human history. The most damaging and critical belief or misunderstanding held by human beings is the idea of separation. The solution is to embrace at last the notion that we are all one."[13]

One day, as we were discussing this, Neale held up his hand with his fingers stretched apart. "Does the fact that my fingers are attached to one hand make them not individual?" he asked, his outstretched hand hovering between us. "The fact that everything is connected does not stop the fingers from being highly individual. Unity does not eliminate individuation." This was a crucial point for me. As I developed gratitude and snapped the rubber band on my wrist in an effort to always choose love, I also sometimes felt a nagging worry that I would be taken advantage of again or once more become overwhelmed by the energetic work I was doing. (Which, as Neale pointed out, meant that I was choosing fear.) But the idea of individuation helped me to understand how to hold oneness in mind *and* establish boundaries.

As I'd started forging more intense energetic bonds with my patients, I had been increasingly struggling to understand where

I stopped and other people started. I needed this crucial reminder that, despite the fact that we're all part of the same thing, we are *not* all the same, that one person might act out of fear while another acts out of love, and that forging psychological and energetic self-protection was necessary. I have since become able to move somewhat fluidly between the transcendent love I feel in the clinic—which is a pure sensation unlike anything I've felt otherwise, not even in my deepest familial intimacies—and the more ordinary, and rugged, interactions of everyday life. One requires a sense of unyielding faith; the other requires a clear view of my needs and a willingness to communicate them honestly.

In *Conversations with God,*[14] there is a moment when God elaborates on how thoughts create a subtle yet influential form of energy. He suggests that once negative thoughts have been put into motion, particularly to the point that they've taken on physical form, such as illness, it takes a shift in perspective to reverse it. This caught my attention because it aligned with the concept of stagnation in Chinese medicine, when energy becomes stuck because of unexpressed or extreme emotion.

While I read, my heart began to beat a little faster, as the words took an even more personal turn for me: "Healers have just such faith," Neale writes. "It is a faith that crosses over into Absolute Knowing. . . . This knowingness is also a thought—and a very powerful one. It has the power to move mountains—to say nothing of molecules in your body."[15] Though this was my third time reading the book, I did not remember this passage. This time, however, since I'd come to view the energy I drew from the universe as a potent force, these words struck me with their depth. I read this passage as a call to arms: I believe that I am able to channel energy from a source that offers the power to heal—it is my privilege and responsibility to avail it to others.

With Neale as a mentor, I had learned a spiritual lesson, but I'd also emerged with a clearer view of what I was tapping into with my energy work and acupuncture. Neale helped me to trust in what I had intuited as a practitioner: that we are in communication with source, this larger energy field, more often than we know. Taking the leap of faith required to believe in this was perhaps the most difficult task for me, but, given my experiences in hospice and with my patients in private practice, I was ready to take it.

Still, keen as ever for more vantage points from which to understand the role of energy in our lives, I reached out to others who'd had similar experiences with this energy as well as those who were studying its existence. I had begun to investigate quantum physics at this point as well. And, just as I was starting to glimpse a larger picture—where the spiritual and scientific begin to fit together—I met Kiran Trace. An old friend from acupuncture school, now a well-respected psychologist and practitioner of Chinese medicine, mentioned Kiran to me, saying that we both had a similar interest in the intersection of science and spirituality. She had been consulting Kiran for advice herself, and thought she might have fresh insights to offer about the function of energy medicine. I trust this friend implicitly, so I contacted Kiran straightaway.

Kiran describes herself as a life coach and teacher, but, for me, she also served as an expressive link between spiritual and scientific interpretations of energy. Though I'd come a distance with Neale and had developed a firm belief in the universal energy field, or source, I was still having difficulty envisioning its broader function in the world. I had a grasp on its function in healing—that much I had experienced for myself—but how did we interact with this source on a daily level? What did that look like? It was such an elusive concept, I found myself struggling to keep it in sight.

Kiran, however, embodies this idea—literally. Let me explain: In 2005, Kiran had an awakening. As she was sitting on her bed, putting on her shoes, she thought, *We never really recognize how beautiful our bodies are—they're so full of light.*[16] It was an odd thought, and she wasn't certain why it had entered her mind, but, as it turned out, it was the last one she would have in her life as she then knew it. When she lifted her eyes, "I looked at the wall and there was no wall, there was no room, by then even the light had disappeared," she told me. "And I was left with just the thought and nothing else."[17]

As she explained to me, "Instead of seeing the wall of my bedroom, all I could see was a choice. I could only see a choice to see this space as a wall. I could see a deep, collective history of choice that this particular space will be seen as 'wall.'"

Kiran believes that in that moment, she lost a kind of filter in her mind and, with it, her sense of being a separate self. "You know how in grade [six] or [seven] we learn that everything is actually made up of atoms?"[18] she writes in her book, *Tools for Sanity.*[19] "An atom is made of an electron that circulates around a neutron, magnetically drawn to the proton inside, and every-thing is made up of these atoms moving through space. Things only appear to be a wall or a table, but actually are made up of vast space filled with moving atoms. I could see the space inside the walls and tables. Things began to appear more quantum to me, more as choices, as potential—potential energy, spaciousness that comes into form."[20] The "potential energy" she describes re-sembles the Tao to me, the emptiness from which the universe flows.

This was not, however, a spiritual revelation for Kiran—"I am a teacher of reality, not spirituality,"[21] she will tell you—it was rather more as if she were suddenly able to see the world in its original emptiness, devoid of form. And it felt so drastic she refers to it as a death. "I remember walking down the street a couple of days after I died,"[22] she writes. "I was watching all this madness unfolding, feeling like the only sober person in a world of crazy drunks . . . I didn't even know how to talk. It felt like every word I uttered was [re-creating] the hell I'd learned to speak from my mistaken identity."[23]

Kiran did eventually learn to assimilate what had happened and the language of this other world. She believes that she is op-erating at the very base level of oneness—which, incidentally, is where she suggests we all operate from but we cannot see past our own identities and egos, or "pain bodies," as Kiran calls them, to realize this. In this new place—"a vast emptiness dreaming itself"—she felt as if she were watching a movie showing an im-age of, say, Brad Pitt and Angelina Jolie driving in a car. "You're sitting in the movie theater, and you know it's only a projection of light casting these images and that there are no actors actually standing in front of you," she explained. "That is the way I realized the world presented itself too."

In my studies of ancient cultures I had learned that South American shamans have long believed that we dream the world into being—so this concept of a projected reality wasn't completely foreign to me. I'd also recently learned from my scientific research that some of the world's leading physicists theorize that our physical reality is a projection—like a hologram—and that what we perceive as three-dimensional reality is stored on a two-dimensional surface at the edge of the universe.

"The idea is similar to that of ordinary holograms where a three-dimensional image is encoded in a two-dimensional surface, such as in the hologram on a credit card,"[24] as Kostas Skenderis, professor of mathematical sciences at the University of Southampton, describes it. "However, this time, the entire universe is encoded."[25] In other words, the seemingly solid world around us, and the dimension of time, are projected from information stored on a flat, 2-D surface.[26]

As you can imagine, this is not an easy hypothesis to prove, but Skenderis was part of a team that provided the first real observational evidence supporting the theory that our universe could be a vast and almost incomprehensibly complex hologram. Researchers from the University of Southampton (UK), University of Waterloo (Canada), Perimeter Institute (Canada), L'Istituto Nazionale di Fisica Nucleare (INFN), Lecce (Italy), and the University of Salento (Italy) published their findings in the journal *Physical Review Letters*.[27] Advances in telescopes and other sensing equipment have allowed scientists to retrieve information hidden in the "white noise" of the universe, also known as the cosmic microwave background, or the afterglow from the Big Bang.

As Skenderis told reporters when his research was published in January 2017, "Holography is a huge leap forward in the way we think about the structure and creation of the universe. Einstein's theory of general relativity explains almost everything large scale in the universe very well, but starts to unravel when examining its origins and mechanisms at quantum level. Scientists have been working for decades to combine Einstein's theory of gravity and quantum theory. Some believe the concept of a holographic universe has the potential to reconcile the two. I hope our research takes us another step [toward] this."[28]

In fact, renowned cosmologist Stephen Hawking's last theory, submitted before his death but published posthumously in *The Journal of High Energy Physics* in March 2018, embraces this idea of a holographic universe, proposing that we are not projecting out of a spatial dimension but we are instead projecting out of the dimension of time from *before* the Big Bang.[29] Hawking, before his death, asserted, "We are not down to a single, unique universe, but . . . a smaller range of possible universes."[30]

If the reality we perceive is more holographic than we understand, then Kiran, like a character from *The Matrix*, is seeing the space behind the illusion. Kiran's experience suggests to me that life emanates from a unified energetic field filled with information. We communicate with this field through our thoughts, feelings, words, and deeds, and in doing so we affect not just our own lives but other people's too.

. . .

Over time, Kiran has not only learned to cope with her unique perspective, but she has also discovered how to use her particular awareness to help others. And though Kiran doesn't describe herself as a healer, I learned a great deal about healing from her.

"This vast, spacious intelligence is not still," Kiran explained. "And when it is moving, it can sometimes assume dense energetic forms, as a wound, as pain, some kind of a pain in our system. We can feel this pain physically, emotionally, and mentally. That pain has a voice, a very aggressive loop in your head, and it tells us all kinds of scary things . . . That is the real reason we experience lack and limitation: because of this constant fear-fueled story in our minds."

Many times in my practice of acupuncture I've witnessed patients overcome by emotion the moment the first needle is inserted. Inevitably, they will say, "I don't know why I'm so upset," as they sob on the table in my little treatment room. I believe that memory doesn't exist solely in our brains but also at a cellular level in our bodies. When my patients were suddenly, inexplicably struck with sorrow during an acupuncture session, it seemed I had tapped an emotional trauma—the "dense energetic form" Kiran described but understood as qi stagnation in Chinese medicine. Upon releasing it, people were, I believe, expressing the pain, emotional and energetic, that had been held there. A 2015 study by researchers at the University of California, Los Angeles, in fact, shows that traces of memory may be stored in a cell's nucleus and can be triggered with a small reminder stimulus, indicating that memories can quite literally be stored in the body.[31]

Kiran takes a different route to find these spots of stagnated energy. She can actually visualize blockage in people's bodies.

"Everybody highlights different things for me and that is how I know what to work on," she told me. "I'll guide them to put their awareness where the obstacle has been created. Maybe I'll get a flash of grief, the challenge between someone and their spouse, for example, but usually the obstacle has roots that are way older than that. We'll trace it together. We'll talk about where that pattern first started, how it got hardwired into their system."

I talk to Kiran regularly. Her unique perspective helped me deal with challenges as my business grew. But, as with every step of this journey, I had to adjust. When I first consulted with Kiran, she informed me that I had blockage in my solar plexus, located in the upper abdomen. She described this as coming from a childhood fear for my survival, but I felt I would have already known if I had blockage there—I was the one, after all, who spent the day revealing this kind of thing to patients. So I politely listened to her tell me she could see this stagnation and then went on with my day. But, later, as I was sitting at home, I thought back to when I was a little girl, curled in the fetal position, my hands clenched at my abdomen, as my mother lashed out. I was instinctively protecting the very area where Kiran had told me I was storing pain. If I had a weak spot, I realized, it was my upper abdomen. I had been plagued by food allergies and digestive problems my whole life. At various times, I've been diagnosed with everything from gallbladder polyps to a hiatal hernia. It dawned on me that these were all ailments located in the solar plexus. Could it be that I *had* stored quite a lot of negative energy in this area of my body? Was there a density there, and would releasing it improve my health?

When I finally surrendered, admitting to Kiran that I thought she was right, she taught me how to move this energy. She taught me to focus on a memory that brought me happiness. I rifled through a series of flashbacks, trying to find something that brought me a sense of warmth and safety, feeling a bit downtrodden at the effort this took—until finally I landed on something. There was a little corner of my childhood house where there was a stained glass window. As a young girl, I would tuck myself away underneath it and, when the sunlight came through, a red beam would cross over me and I would curl up in its light. With Kiran's instructions, I remembered the warmth and consolation of this red beam, and then I imagined it going into my solar plexus. And I pictured the warm consoling energy meeting the density of the pain and the knot began unraveling. The changes were imperceptible at first, but over time my abdominal discomfort receded into the background and then one day I realized I couldn't feel it so acutely anymore.

What Kiran taught me—something I frankly should have already known from my work as an acupuncturist—is that you can't move stuck energy with force or coercion. You can only move it with tenderness and love. And Kiran believes—similar to Neale's notion of choosing fear over love—that it is human nature to more instinctively attach to our pain rather than our happiness. Both Kiran and Neale maintain that source responds to these choices and the energy that results.

Kiran now exists without a "separate from everybody else" self. She has more access to choice, to spaciousness, to the connected field of unity that sounds like the peace and immersive light described by my hospice patients. I understand this on an intellectual level, and I can feel that ease and peace when talking with her, even if I can't always live it. But I can access it in my healing work.

When I pair my spiritual perspective with science, however, I feel more of a sense of understanding about both energy healing and life itself. Where spirituality assumes that the world is vast and infinite, science seeks to define and limit, to discern only that which is measurable—ultimately, however, they are both reaching for the same thing. They are both attempting to fathom the universe.

YOU THE HEALER

Grounding and Opening

Some healers use rituals to protect themselves from energy that they consider to be negative. To me this has always seemed to reflect an underlying fear (which is more likely to cause restriction and contraction). This exercise is intended to help you ground and open your body in order to tap into the vast matrix of intelligence in the field around and within you—a field that I call source but that could equally be referred to as God or the Tao. Source flows through you, so you are never separated from it, though it may sometimes feel as if you are. This visualization helps to strengthen the connection.

- Stand with your feet shoulder width apart and your arms by your sides. Bend your knees slightly and shift your weight until you feel steady.
- Tilt your pelvis forward slightly and straighten your spine.

- Shift your awareness to the base of your spine and imagine a cord of energy, like a laser beam, traveling from the base of the spine deep into the earth. Feel your feet on the floor and notice that you feel subtly heavier and more grounded.
- Imagine a ball of bright light above you and then visualize that light entering your body through the top of your head. Feel the light filling your body, extending through your trunk and into your limbs.

As you practice this exercise, you may start to feel your connection to source energy. And, in my experience, the more you practice the more you will experience this energy as intelligent. For example, these days, if I lose my keys (which I seem to do regularly), I slip into this posture, ground, connect, and ask for guidance. I invariably find my keys moments later.

4

INTO THE LAB

On a gorgeous early summer day in 2017, Bill Bengston, a professor of sociology at St. Joseph's College, ascended the stage of a Yale auditorium and introduced eighty-seven-year-old physicist Robert Jahn—a bit frail but no less deterred from his mission. The audience received him warmly and with admiration: Jahn was a giant in their field. (Sadly, Jahn would pass away just five months after this event.) I was at the thirty-sixth annual conference for the Society for Scientific Exploration (SSE), held on this occasion at Yale University. An assorted group of scientists, physicists, psychiatrists, engineers, and philosophers had gathered— united by their interest in peer-reviewed science pushed beyond conventional boundaries. There had been presentations on coincidence, phantom limb pain, and out-of-body experiences. This being academia, however, sober titles held their eccentric subjects in check: *Dogma, Heresy, and the Religion of Science: Is it Time for a Reformation of Empiricism?*; *A Multi-Frequency Replication of the MegaREG Experiments; An Emerging New Paradigm for Complementary Medicine.*[1]

The crowd was largely composed of professors and researchers who had, at great professional risk, diverged from established scholarly paths to explore the esoteric world. (A standard piece of advice doled out by senior SSE members to younger academics with a bent toward the mystical: "Get tenure first!") These people, trained to gather analytic evidence in support of their theories, have brought the rigors of science and research to bear on such topics as ESP, entanglement, and energy healing. It is a contrary combination—like trying to fill a beaker with intuition—and, as such, it is the path of most resistance within the hallowed walls of academia.

Here at the SSE conference, though, these radical academics were among their own. The audience stood in appreciation for Jahn, who'd himself endured the suspicions of many of his peers at Princeton while pioneering the "anomalous" research—as SSE-ers describe their work—that had inspired many of the people gathered in the room. Bengston, standing alongside Jahn onstage, would later give a presentation of his own—*The Reverse Engineering Healing Project*—studiously detailing experiments in which mice were injected with mammary cancer and then healed with a hands-on energy technique. It takes a steely armor to build these careers, doggedly pursuing research in the laboratory that is reflexively shunned by conventional science. This was Jahn's moment of honor, but he was also passing the baton: in Bengston, he'd found a stalwart, a mystic visionary with a scientist's curiosity, forging ahead in his experimental work with a sharp focus on healing.

Bengston possesses an emphatic matter-of-factness, almost studiously so, as if to gird himself against the inevitable prejudices. He is practical about—and sometimes amused by—the elusive nature of healing in general. "The take-home message is that we're making it all up," he instructs, smiling impishly, while teaching his course, the Bengston Energy Healing Method. "It's just like going for a medical opinion and they say 'get a second opinion.' Well what does that mean? We're making it up. Conventional medicine is often a series of best guesses. Very little is known about conventional healing *and* unconventional healing. Different people will tell you different things. Question them all." He isn't looking for God or glory or fortune (he once healed a man of neck cancer, he says, in exchange for a homegrown zucchini)—but, as with everyone else I've met along this way, he is gripped. Over the course of his four-decade career, he claims to have not only successfully treated mice (in the lab) but also humans (in life) with various types of cancer—bone, breast, brain, and pancreatic among them—as well as a wide variety of other less severe illnesses. (I spoke with a sixty-eight-year-old woman who'd been treated by Bill—she'd met him through her husband, a family medicine doctor—for stage-IIB pancreatic cancer. Though her prognosis was that she would live only a few more months, she has been cancer-free for nearly a year.) More than anything, Bill Bengston wants to know *how* this happens.

I first met Bill through Kell Julliard, then the head of research at NYU Lutheran Medical Center (now called NYU Langone Hospital–Brooklyn) in 2014. I'd founded an acupuncture program at the labor and delivery wing of the hospital a decade earlier and had stayed in touch with Kell afterward. When I mentioned to him that I'd been looking into the empirical research behind healing—that is, efforts made in a lab to investigate what occurs during this process—he immediately suggested that I meet a professor he knew who'd been healing mice with cancer. As it turned out, I'd already read about this astounding work in a book called *The Energy Cure: Unraveling the Mystery of Hands-On Healing*[2]—written by none other than Bill Bengston. The next week, Kell introduced me to Bill in person at a dinner in Brooklyn.

Bill, a studious-looking man in glasses, button-down oxford, and khakis, is fascinating and funny and irreverent. He is an old-school eccentric, with a refreshingly frank demeanor, free of self-aggrandizement or phoniness. The healing business is riddled with fraudulent characters (we'll get to them in Chapter 9), but Bill is as deliberate as the best scientists. In fact, he is as startled by his own findings as the best scientists: He continues to be stunned by his own extraordinary results in the lab. And his theories about what might be happening—the transfer of information that takes place between healer and patient—are persuasive. I felt I'd met a fellow traveler on a familiar journey.

In 1971, when Bengston was a twenty-one-year-old living with his parents in Great Douglaston, Long Island, making ends meet by working as a lifeguard at a local pool, he met a forty-eight-year-old man named Bennett Mayrick. Another lifeguard had pointed Mayrick out one afternoon, mockingly describing him as a "psychic." Bengston's attitude then—"I was open-minded to psychic phenomenon in principle,"[3] he writes, "but intensely skeptical of those claiming to produce it"—is essentially the same today. And yet, then as now, he was curious enough to find out what this extrasensory skill truly entailed. So he introduced himself.

In their first meeting, Mayrick managed to impress Bengston— among other feats, he was able to accurately intuit things about Bengston's life by holding his wallet in the palm of his hand. "When I hold an object," Mayrick confided, "I get an urge to say something, but I don't know what until I hear myself say it."[4] Mayrick's unusual ability and his ambivalence about it—he seemed "both excited and threatened" by what he could do— appealed to Bengston.

Soon the two men were in business together, albeit in an un-expected way. Mayrick made his living as a maid and enlisted Bengston to be his cleaning partner. (Simultaneously, Bengston studied for, and later received, a master's degree in sociology at St. John's University.) But it was through this alliance that Bengston was able to persuade Mayrick to take a more official view of his psychic abilities. He discovered Mayrick possessed an ability to attune to other people's pain—first revealed when Mayrick picked up a letter and suddenly got a terrible headache; meanwhile, the person who'd sent the letter, when contacted, explained she was suffering a migraine. When Mayrick concentrated on making his own headache go away—by imagining the pain dissolving— the woman, too, felt her migraine lift. Intrigued, Bengston urged Mayrick to treat his chronic lower back pain. When Mayrick put his hand to the small of Bengston's back, there was an immedi-ate sensation of warmth. "As the heat penetrated my spine, I felt my lower back grow numb in a four-inch radius, as if shot with Novocain,"[5] Bengston explains. "With Ben's hand still on my back, the numbness wore off from the outer edges in. When he removed his hand, the last spot of numbness disappeared." The whole thing lasted ten minutes, and Bengston has not felt pain in his back since.

Mayrick was persuaded enough to practice healing on friends and acquaintances; Bengston was curious enough to study what was happening in search of a pragmatic explanation. He witnessed many strange and wonderful scenes between Mayrick and the people he healed—one person regained partial vision, another's hearing was restored, one woman's gangrene disappeared just days before she was scheduled to have her infected foot amputated, and, finally, after Mayrick grew more accustomed to his talent, he successfully treated a variety of cancers. Throughout, Bengston played the office manager and analyst, keeping the practice organized while attempting to decipher what transpired when Mayrick healed.

Of the many things that fascinated Bengston about the peculiar ins and outs of these encounters, he was most confounded by the restless reaction some had when they underwent a healing. "Many who entered the 'hocus-pocus' world of hands-on healing seemed geared to expect instantaneous cures as validation," Bengston points out, "quite unlike the frustrations they were willing to endure within the traditional medical system."[6] Many patients who improved after one treatment but weren't yet fully recovered, in fact didn't return. But the procedure was noninvasive, involving no risk—making it a nothing-to-lose prospect—so why did it spook or offend them?

This was not faith-based healing. There was no sense, on Mayrick's part, that he was working in service of a greater spiritual being; he preferred, in fact, that his patients not bring faith, or even expectation, to the transaction. The only belief that Mayrick held about what he was able to do was that he was harnessing some kind of energy at large in the world, available to us all. Mayrick's attitude about the healing process was so utilitarian, he believed it could be taught to anyone.

A year into practicing, Mayrick encouraged Bengston to try to heal alongside him, insisting that he'd not only felt Bengston generating an energy during the sessions, but he'd been drawing on it too. Reluctantly, Bengston started treating small pains and ailments. When he did, he felt, as Mayrick had, a surge of energy and his hands heated up as he held them on a patient's body. Bengston, practical by nature, was convinced—if he could do this, it must not be supernatural. At about the same time, Mayrick decided to start teaching his patients how to heal too. He wanted those he worked with to take a more active role in the partnership, so that they understood what was happening when he worked with them. Perhaps, too, he wanted to share in the responsibility of something so intangible but with such significant outcomes.

Mayrick and Bengston became determined to prove that this type of healing was not the result of being extraordinarily empathic, or "touched" in some way, but rather a practical, cultivated skill. In their analysis, they discovered that one of the most crucial components to successful healing was for the practitioner to remain detached during the treatment. Mayrick described it as continuously "distracting his mind from his hands" so that the energy would not be impeded by intellect or ego. (Not unlike my own need to divert my attention while in clinic.) Mayrick and Bengston, believing that this energy channeling worked both ways, devised a method by which the patients, too, could learn to distract themselves from the afflictions they so fervently wanted to heal.

The two men instructed patients to engage in "cycling,"[7] which requires devising a mental Rolodex of twenty images with no connection to healing. These images are meant to represent personal desires—objects, honors, physical or psychological yearnings. They should be viewed as wishes fulfilled—that is, as if they were already a reality. This Rolodex of desire is meant to feed the ego in order to get it out of the way. Their theory was that one should be selfish while practicing: cycling is about thinking about what you want rather than putting yourself in a position of selflessness.

"Selflessness builds resentment," Bengston would later explain when I took his course, by which he means that if a healer believes he is practicing only for others, as a complete sacrifice, there is a temptation to be a martyr. But healing extends out of enthusiasm and joy; we are not open to the energy otherwise. I've found, in my own practice, that the energy comes more freely with a frank acceptance of my interwoven motivations. Of course I want to heal others, *and* of course I feel good about myself when I do. "Thank the healee," advises Bengston, tipping his students' mental states toward gratitude. "They're giving *you* what you want."[8]

As a person is able to flash through these images more quickly—ideally, achieving a state in which they run through the mind so fast as to blur—he or she becomes more able to give and receive energy. As Bill once aptly described it: "Healing is an autonomic"—meaning unconscious—"response to need."[9] If the person's mind is occupied by something else—such as a flashing image of a beach house, which, incidentally, is one of the visuals I used when I tried cycling—then they won't be concentrating on the healing. And if they're not concentrating on healing, it will happen naturally—"as an autonomic response to need." (Later, Bengston would conduct a study designed to test this theory: While in an fMRI machine, he had a technician put a series of envelopes in his hand. Some were empty; some contained strands of hair of dogs with cancer [supplied by a veterinarian]. Without his knowing which envelope was being placed in his hand, the MRI showed his brain reacted in a dramatically different way when he came into contact with the hair of a dog with cancer—and, therefore, in need.)[10]

The notions that healing could be taught, and that cycling was the way to learn, would become cornerstones of Bengston's work going forward. Bengston went on to refine the cycling technique, and he would soon bring these to bear in the laboratory—without Mayrick—in an investigation of the healing process. As Bengston became more pragmatic in his drive to understand healing, Mayrick began to drift into a darker emotional state, growing more reliant on teaching as a way to prop up his own beliefs. He became increasingly resistant to Bengston's efforts to understand what was happening in a clinical way.

As the distance grew between the two men, Bengston met David Krinsley, who'd participated in Mayrick's group lessons for a brief period. Krinsley was a geology professor from Queens College of the City University of New York. He had written hundreds of scientific papers, including cover stories for *Science*[11] and *Nature*[12] magazines, which especially piqued Bengston's interest, as these are the most prestigious publications in the field. He also shared Bengston's ambition to explore healing in the lab. Fortunately, Krinsley had also once served as an interim provost at Queens College, giving him broad access to the institution; he was able to persuade the chairman of the biology department to allow them to conduct an experiment of their own design under the aegis of the university.

A researcher in the biology department would provide twelve mice injected with a particular strain of mammary cancer—six would undergo hands-on healing on a daily basis; the other six would remain with the researcher as a control group. Mice injected with this type of cancer of the mammary glands, by all scientific research accounts, resulted in 100 percent fatality between fourteen to twenty-seven days.[13] So, if any of the mice recovered, it would be of scientific note.

Krinsley assigned Bengston the task of healing during the experiment. After an early panic that he wouldn't be able to perform, Bengston engaged the cycling method he'd been teaching others. As he did, with hands placed on either side of the cage, he felt his left hand heat up and then "the beginning of a current" started to pass through him. Over time, Bengston became so adept at achieving the state he needed to be in that, on occasion, he became completely unburdened. "The detachment I felt from my hands, then my entire body, coalesced into a sense of oneness with the mice," Bengston writes of the experience. "All my doubts about the healings seemed trivial, and I was pervaded with peace and well-being. My mind emptied of thought. I simply was."[14]

Bengston treated the mice for an hour every day and, after

just over a week, they developed tumors large enough to deform their bodies. Bengston declared the experiment a failure. Krinsley objected, remarking that, despite their physical appearances, the mice were moving about the cage normally. Bengston pressed on. Small blackened spots, "like pencil points,"[15] appeared on the tumors. Bengston begged Krinsley to end the project; he was despondent watching the mice suffer. Krinsley encouraged him with the news that if a single mouse lived past twenty-seven days, it would be a scientific phenomenon. The biology researcher who'd been working with these same mice for the last twenty years, after all, hadn't yet found a way to make them survive that long, much less achieve remission.

Shortly thereafter, the tumors on the mice Bengston had treated began to ulcerate, blooming into weeping red wounds. It seemed another blow—except that the mice were continuing to scramble about as if nothing was wrong. The twenty-eighth day came and went, and the mice were still alive. Then the ulcerations turned from red to white; the tumors began to shrink. The mice's fur grew back. It was as if time were improbably turning backward until, finally, the mice looked the same as the day the experiment had begun. When the biologist who'd injected the mice tested them, all of the mice were cancer-free.

It was such overwhelming news—challenging every conventional notion they'd ever held—it left them literally speechless. Both men had to take a break from each other—and the work— for several weeks. When they came back to the lab, they committed to replicating the experiment. They also received a startling addendum to the results of their last test: the four remaining control mice had also gone into remission.[16]

Bengston and Krinsley conducted four more healing experiments with cancer-injected mice, with some changes in design. For one, Bengston stepped back as the healer, focusing solely on the research, replacing himself first with Krinsley and then with the chairs of the biology departments of the two colleges where they conducted the experiments—Queens College and St. Joseph's College—as well as small groups of students, none of whom believed in hands-on healing. "I wouldn't take a student who wasn't skeptical," says Bengston in his characteristic no-nonsense tone. "Believers scare me. They spend too much time defending their own beliefs rather than trying to figure out what is going on."[17] For each of the experiments, Bengston taught the participants the cycling method. He also added a second control group of mice that were shipped off campus.

Forty-eight mice were subjected to healing overall—combining the mice treated in all the experiments—out of which, forty-four were healed. Of the combined control mice in the first group—those that were left on campus—thirty-three out of forty-one went into remission. And of the last group, the mice sent off campus for the duration of the experiment, none survived.[18]

Bengston knew that they'd achieved something incredible—87.9 percent of the treated mice had returned to their healthy states, which, by even the most rational assessment, suggested they had been healed by the hands-on method rather than spontaneous remission—but he couldn't make sense of the control mice. Why had such a large number of the first control group recovered while none of the second control group did?

Bengston didn't yet have an answer for that question, but he wanted to publish the findings right away. He and Krinsley sent their research to *Science* and *Nature*, where Krinsley had published before. They learned, however, that neither magazine would even send out their findings for peer review. "They don't do those kinds of papers," Bengston recalls learning. "It was almost a statement of pride for them. They only do 'real' things."

Ultimately, in 2000, Bengston and Krinsley did publish their study, "The Effect of the 'Laying On of Hands' on Transplanted Breast Cancer in Mice," in the *Journal of Scientific Exploration*.[19]

Bengston decided to take a break from the unorthodox path he'd been pursuing, which turned into quite an extended leave. After a couple of decades of ruminating—during which he returned to the more conventional world of sociology, first getting his PhD at Fordham University and then teaching the sociology of religion as well as research methods and statistics at St. Joseph's College—Bengston was struck with an idea about why the first group of control mice went into remission.

"This was my eureka insight: spatial separation doesn't always mean independence,"[20] Bengston recalls. "Though the treated and control mice were kept in different locations, something unseen must have continued to connect them so that whatever happened to the treated mice also happened to most of the control mice." The majority of the mice in the first control group, he reasoned, became part of what he calls "resonant bonding,"[21] or what some researchers, based on a theory put forth more recently by Kings College psychology professor Imants Barušs, now call a "meaning field."[22] That is, the control mice that went into remission were able to do so because they were brought into a dynamic field of energy and intent created by the healer-researchers. In every experiment, someone grew curious about

how the first group of control mice were faring, and broke protocol, visiting them in the separate room where they were being
kept. Bengston did in the first experiment; the head of the biology department did in the next one; and the students who participated as healers did in the rest. Nobody, however, who took
part in the experiments that included a second control group of
mice, those that were sent off campus, came into contact with
them. And all of the mice from this group died.

"In the same way that you can experience connection and disconnection subjectively," Bengston theorizes, "you can also experience connection and disconnection experimentally."[23] The first
control group had been included in a healing bond—perhaps
through the healers bringing them into their consciousness—
whereas the second control group had been excluded. "You can
construct and deconstruct resonant bonds through consciousness," Bengston concludes. "But the question remains: *How* does
this happen?"[24]

Bengston thinks of meaning fields as an extension, or an off-
shoot, of something called morphic field theory[25] posited by biologist and philosopher Rupert Sheldrake. This theory suggests
that the forms of self-organizing living things—everything from
molecules to people to entire galaxies—are shaped by a cumula-
tive and collective memory spanning generations; information is
passed down as imprints within the larger energy field. Put more
plainly, Sheldrake believes that humans, as a species, along with
animals and plants, "remember" how to act based on the behavior of prior generations, a process he calls "morphic resonance."[26]

"Sheldrake would predict if you put out a healing field [or
meaning field], then *all* the mice within the sphere of influence

of that field would be affected," says Bengston, "but in my case, I've got control mice that are not affected. I think that Sheldrake's idea of morphic resonance is wonderful, but it's incomplete.[27] There needs to be something that you loosely switch on to create the resonant bond." By "loosely," he means in passing; for example, when I create a resonant bond with my patients, it doesn't tend to last longer than when we are in the treatment room together; such a bond can be turned on and off fairly easily. Bengston believes we can form similar bonds en masse, and this can affect the entire group, as it did with the control mice in his experiments. Bengston has since replicated this experiment with cancerous mice eleven more times, all with the same results. (And, in so doing, has discovered that he consistently feels the healing energy from his left hand. What's more, the sick mice gravitated to that hand instinctively every time.)

As an undergraduate student, before Bengston had even met Mayrick, he'd discovered the work of Dr. Bernard Grad, a research oncologist at McGill University in Toronto. The researcher, in large part, inspired Bengston's career. Grad—or "the Great Grad," as Bengston likes to call him—was also determined to bring energy healing out of the realm of the abstract and into the exacting world of science. During the sixties and seventies, Grad extensively tested Oskar Estebany, an uneducated Hungarian man who ostensibly cured through hands-on healing. Estebany had realized his talent while in the Hungarian cavalry—when he would pet sick horses, they would become healthy again. Estebany did not claim to be a healer—in fact, he insisted he was simply petting the horses and had no idea why others found what he did noteworthy. He did, however, allow Grad to test him in the laboratory.[28]

In one experiment similar to the one Bengston would himself later do, Grad divided surgically wounded mice into two groups, one to be treated by Estebany and one to be a control group. Estebany held the cages of his mice for fifteen minutes, twice a day, for the duration of the experiment. In the end, Estebany's mice healed more quickly than the control group.[29]

Next, Grad wanted to test if Estebany's hands generated an energy that could charge other substances. Grad exposed some goiter-induced mice to scraps of cotton and wool that Estebany had treated by holding it for a time, while a control group was exposed to untouched scraps. The mice who came into contact with the treated scraps showed a significantly slower rate of goiter formation, suggesting that Estebany's hands had transmitted energy into the material.

Inspired by Grad and Estebany, Bengston also tried transferring energy to cotton. He once gave cotton he'd charged—by walking around with it in his hands as he cycled—to a woman he knew with ductal carcinoma, a form of breast cancer. First, he'd done a hands-on treatment with her in person, but then, because she lived a long distance away, he gave her the cotton to treat herself. A year after her cancer had been deemed to be in remission by her doctor, Bengston visited her at her home. She asked if he would charge some more material for her, to be on the safe side, and handed him a piece of cotton. Immediately, Bengston felt a pain in his armpit. When he put his hand there, he felt a small lump. When he pressed the woman as to why this might be, she disclosed that this was the cotton that had been previously charged by him—and she'd slept with it when she was still sick. "I think there is a memory in the cotton," Bengston explains. "I think it takes on the thing it was used for."[30] Now, Bill instructs everyone he teaches to discard all cotton after a week's use. And, though Bengston considers himself strictly a researcher and only heals friends or family members if they make a special request, he does heal *himself* with cotton from time to time. (Incidentally, when I took Bengston's healing course, I asked my researcher on this book to come along with me. He agreed to do it, but he was dubious, to say the least. Still, he charged his own cotton, as we all did in the course, and then dutifully slept with it taped to his bad back. A week later, he confessed, with good-natured outrage, that his back felt "stupidly better.")

Bengston designed a study to investigate this phenomenon. At Brown University, Bengston and his researchers placed charged cotton and uncharged cotton near puncture wounds in cells and found that the cells genomically respond to the cotton that has been charged. "If they have motility," Bengston adds, "they will actually swim toward the cotton like the mice moved toward my left hand."[31]

Throughout history, almost all religious traditions have incorporated the notion that objects can be infused with powers that heal or protect people. The Christian concept of holy water is one of the earliest examples of this. (Not one to leave a research stone unturned, Bengston has also explored the possibility of putting energy into water in the lab. In a study conducted at the University of Connecticut, he charged water and then treated cancer-injected mice with it, resulting in the mice going into remission.)

Native Americans and other indigenous groups have also long believed that crystals and minerals generate healing energy and that skilled shamans can manipulate them to generate specific patterns of frequencies for healing.

My own mother, when she was nearly on her deathbed with cancer, relied heavily on a small metal charm, given to her by a colleague of mine from acupuncture school. My friend was a devout Buddhist who had spent many years in India and Nepal; when she gave the charm to my mother, she told her it had been blessed by the Dalai Lama. It brought my mother great comfort. She held it as she endured chemotherapy, and I found it next to her bed when she died. Of course, it didn't save her life, but did it have a restorative energy? Certainly my mother, who had no connection to Buddhism or the Dalai Lama, drew a kind of protective strength from her amulet—and Bengston's studies would back her up.

Once Bengston was able to effectively charge cotton and water, he wanted to push the boundaries a bit further. More recently, he has begun to charge cell medium—putting in what he has come to call "information,"[32] his preferred term for energy in these experiments, since it seems whatever he is drawing can be transferred to an inanimate object—and found that when he put cancerous cells into that medium, the cancerous tissue itself was changed in nine measurable ways.

Ultimately, Bengston speculates that energy—or information—is "piggybacking"[33] on a wave frequency. If, indeed, this is true, then the information he uses to heal should be able to find a frequency through any source. As such, Bengston has begun doing sound recordings when he charges cotton and testing them in the Brown University laboratory, funded by Emerald Gate Charitable Trust, to see if they, too, can effect a change. "So far we have looked at 167 cancer genes," Bengston says. "If you play this recording . . . a good chunk of the genes genomically change. And this is a reliable effect. Overall, we have seen genomic changes in cancer whether you do it live with your hands, use cotton, or whether you do it with this recording. We're affecting telomere length and inflammation and immunology. And we're starting to understand the mechanism by which cancer is cured."[34]

Bengston asserts—and aims for his research to corroborate this—that all three healing methods (hands-on, charged cotton, recordings) are creating apoptosis, the death of a cell that occurs as a normal part of an organism's growth. This is vital in the case of cancer—which causes cells to grow uncontrollably rather than die. (It is interesting to note, then, that Bengston maintains that he is not able to heal people with cancers that have been treated with radiation or chemotherapy because, he believes, the information cannot affect a damaged cell. On the other hand, Bengston points out that he has students who, after learning his healing method, report that they *have* successfully treated people who've undergone radiation and chemo.) Of course, Bengston's ambitions don't stop there: next, he hopes to develop an app that will deliver a healing frequency from your iPhone.

I have spent a great deal of time considering Bengston's work. I've reviewed his research, read his book, and taken his course; I've interviewed him for countless hours. Eventually I realized, for all of his scientific rigor and forward-thinking ideas, he'd actually, in a way, led me back with more confidence to my early instinct, and the ancient Chinese belief that the needles of acupuncture are like little antennae, picking up curative information from the energy field around us.

YOU THE HEALER

Rapid Image Cycling

Bengston and Mayrick stumbled upon an unusual method to distract the healer's ego in order to allow information to flow between a healer and patient. Here is the method Bengston taught to those participating in lab-based mouse studies. A fuller explanation is available in the *Journal of Alternative and Complementary Medicine.*[35]

Make a list of at least twenty things you want, without worrying about how and when these wishes might be realized. This list can encompass material things, health matters, states of mind, or situations involving other people (though as a matter of ethics you should not include another person without their knowledge and consent).

Visualize each item on the list with an image of the wish having been accomplished. Memorize these images so that you can recall them without effort (this can take some time).

Once you have memorized the images, practice cycling them rapidly in your mind until this becomes so effortless that you can perform other tasks while doing it. Bill finds that experienced "cyclers" can flash at least twenty-four images per second through their minds, but this does take some practice. I imagine my images on a filmstrip and then run it as quickly as I can, all the while seeing rapidly changing images on a screen in my mind's eye.

Once you are comfortable with the image cycling technique, you can experiment with image cycling while placing your hands on or directly above a partner. In Bill's experience, both the healer and the "patient" feel energy or heat emanating from the healer's left hand.

5

MOVING THE NEEDLE

In 1996, scientists at the Roslin Institute in Edinburgh, Scotland, were keeping a radical project under wraps. Unbeknownst to the rest of the world, including their colleagues in the scientific community, they were attempting to clone a sheep. Their plan was simple—or so they thought. First, the team removed an unfertilized egg from an adult female sheep and extracted its DNA. Thanks to a process called meiosis, the DNA of an egg is incomplete, which allows it to combine with the DNA of a sperm to create an embryo. In lieu of sperm, however, the researchers removed the egg's incomplete DNA and replaced it with a full set of DNA taken from a cell of that same adult female sheep's body.

And then the researchers hit a wall. The DNA from a mature cell is technically complete, but it has also lost some of its capacity. As it ages, an adult cell turns on parts of its DNA, whatever is needed to fulfill specific functions—such as creating a bone or even a freckle—and then switches them off again once the tasks are complete. The scientists in Edinburgh realized that they had the ingredients for creating life within their grasp, if only they could unlock this cell's potential, making it behave as if it were young again. In an inspired move—and employing a somewhat *Frankenstein*-like concept—they introduced a tiny electric charge into the process. Amazingly, this was the spark needed to bring the egg to life. Thus Dolly the sheep, the first mammal ever to be cloned from the cell of an adult animal—and our first ovine celebrity—was introduced to the world in 1997.

I was a student at Chinese medical school at the time, and the news intrigued me. The idea that electricity was the impetus needed to produce life struck me as meaningful: an electrical energy that was a vital animating source sounded a lot like the Chinese concept of qi to me.

The idea that the body has electrical properties dates back to 1789, when an Italian physicist, Luigi Galvani, made a discovery while dissecting a dead frog. He touched the frog's exposed sciatic nerve with a charged metal scalpel and noticed that the leg flexed as if the frog were alive. (The word, "galvanize"— meaning to stimulate, or stir to life, with electricity—came into being as a tribute to Galvani.) Two years later, he reported these findings in an academic journal, *Proceedings of the Bologna Academy*;[1] out of this simple observation grew the modern field of bioelectromagnetism, the study of electrical and electromagnetic phenomena—such as the electric currents that flow in our nerves and muscles—that are crucial to our body's ability to function.

When looking at human physiology, the basic unit of bioelectromagnetism is the cell. Most types of cells exhibit some form of polarity, which means that there is an electrical difference across the cell membrane, creating a voltage gradient—also called an electric potential. Some cells, including neurons and muscle cells, have particularly high electrical potential due to electrically excitable membranes whose purpose it is to transmit the electrical impulses that send signals around our bodies.

Qi is not unlike this electrical activity in that it, too, is invisible and understood mostly by its effect. But there is this distinguishing factor: science believes in one and not the other. That may be because the concept of qi, to scientists, can seem too abstract. The word is often translated into English as "energy," although qi doesn't really correlate to the scientific definition of energy. The literal translation of qi is "breath" or "air," and the Chinese character represents the vapor that rises from a pan of rice, signifying the way food becomes energy. But, as I've discussed throughout, qi is also far more than this. Qi is the body's intelligence and its organizing system—and it links us to the greater field of the Tao.

When I was part of the acupuncture program in the labor and delivery wing of Lutheran Medical Center, I learned an important lesson about qi as it translates to the body's electrical energy. For two years, in addition to running my private practice, I ran Lutheran's inpatient acupuncture services, where part of my job was to deliver care to women in labor. My primarily low-income patients often arrived with many challenges and few resources. When things got down to the excruciating nitty-gritty, as they inevitably do in labor, it was very gratifying to be able to offer these women a respite. Sometimes the pain was so intense and chaotic, they were hardly even aware of the needles going in, but they certainly took notice once the pain abated.

To make that happen, I would insert a needle in an acupuncture point known as "Spleen 6," which is about three fingers' breadth up from the medial malleolus, the knob-like bone of the ankle. Spleen 6 is a crossing point of three acupuncture channels, all of which affect the reproductive organs, and because of this it is used to calm uterine pain and menstrual cramps as well as speed up labor. Once I had the needle in, I would "put some qi on it," as I like to say, which meant stimulating it by twisting it slightly with my fingers for about a minute. I knew that I was done when I would feel the needle grab—that is, I would feel a tug, almost like a fish taking the bait. The Chinese call this sensation *de qi*; patients can feel it on their end, too, sometimes as a tingling or deep ache around the needle. It was in doing this, time and again for these women in urgent need of a remedy, that I came to realize that the needle grab was essential.

When I did feel that satisfying little tug, the pain would not only begin to ease more readily, but these women's cervixes would also dilate more quickly—there were midwives, nurses, and doctors examining them after the treatment to confirm this. I was also overseeing acupuncture students in this program, so, once I'd established that this made all the difference, I began to watch like a hawk to be sure my students were getting the needle grab too. I could actually see from the door of a hospital room if one of my students had only superficially inserted a needle, leaving it listing to one side, or if they had established this more profound relationship. "Fewer needles," I remember frequently calling out. "More *de qi*!"

The effect was so pronounced, in fact, that one of the doctors overseeing labor and delivery suggested that we chart what we were doing with patients on the contraction printouts. (Yes, there were still printouts then.) We began to write down on the contractions graphs when we'd treated with acupuncture, at what point we felt the needle grab, and the effect on the patient. In doing so, we created a clear record that treating the Spleen 6 point, when accompanied by a strong needle sensation, increased contraction strength and frequency in addition to dilating the cervix more quickly.

It is always a relief to have instinctual practices verified in a concrete way, and yet, despite the fact that we'd been able to track the success of the *de qi* sensation at this acupuncture point, I still didn't have a clear idea of what was occurring internally. That is, not until nearly a decade later, when I came across new research that specifically investigated this phenomenon and the physiological effect it has on the body.

Helene M. Langevin,[2] a clinical endocrinologist who was curious enough about her patients' interest in acupuncture that she took a course in Chinese medicine and then carried her newfound skills into the lab with her at the department of neurology at the University of Vermont College of Medicine, led a study that found[3] a measurable "pull out force" after every needle grab. And the strength of this grab was, on average, 18 percent higher when measured at acupuncture points as opposed to nonacupuncture points. This was, to me, a corroboration of the anatomy as designed by Chinese medicine; the needle grab is more vigorous at these points because they are more conductive of electrical energy.

Perhaps more crucially, however, Langevin and her colleagues found, experimenting with acupuncture on a piece of rat abdominal wall, that when they rotated the needles—putting some qi on them—the connective tissue underneath the skin became "mechanically attached." Writes Langevin: "Even a small amount of rotation caused the connective tissue to wrap around the needle, like spaghetti winding around a fork."[4] Langevin also found that the tissue remains stretched in this way for the duration of the acupuncture treatment, causing chemical changes at a cellular level that increase electrical conductivity.[5]

Connective tissue, long underplayed by Western medicine and science, has recently become of interest, particularly among molecular and physiological researchers, as new evidence has demonstrated that such stimulation to the connective tissue can be sensed at a cellular level, decreasing chronic inflammation, reducing pain, and even potentially inhibiting the growth of cancer cells or fibrotic tissue.

Connective tissue is everywhere inside of us—"one could draw a line between any two points of the body via a path of connective tissue,"[6] Langevin points out. And it has many functions: it holds organs in place, offers a path for nerves and blood vessels, stores energy and attaches muscle to bone, and, yes, conducts electricity. The latter ability is thanks to a critical component of connective tissue: collagen. There are layers of water bound to collagen fibers that form a uniquely conductive pathway, allowing an electrical charge to travel rapidly throughout the body, just as it did when Dolly the cloned sheep was suddenly brought to life.

I felt vindicated in a new way when I discovered this research. *I was feeling qi in the needle grab*, I thought. And it was not only activating the connective tissue but also conducting electrical energy, sending a message of relief throughout the bodies of those women at Lutheran, allowing them to relax, at least for a little while, as they entered motherhood.

Richard Nixon, of all people, had a hand in introducing acupuncture to America. Before Nixon made his famous visit to China in 1972—allowing Americans to glimpse the country for the first time in more than two decades (since the Communist party assumed power in 1949)—National Security Advisor Henry Kissinger traveled there to pave the way for the upcoming presidential visit. James Reston, a reporter for the *New York Times,* was also in China as part of the advance team before Nixon's visit. Soon after arriving, however, Reston found himself in need of an emergency appendectomy. After having undergone this procedure in a hospital in Beijing, he began to feel serious discomfort while in recovery. "Li Chang-yuan, doctor of acupuncture at the hospital, with my approval, inserted three long, thin needles into the outer part of my right elbow and below my knees and manipulated them in order to stimulate the intestine and relieve the pressure and distension of the stomach,"[7] Reston wrote in his front-page *New York Times* article chronicling his surprise introduction to traditional Chinese medicine. "Meanwhile, Doctor Li lit two pieces of an herb called ai [ye], which looked like the burning stumps of a broken cheap cigar, and held them close to my abdomen while occasionally twirling the needles into action." Reston went on to confide that he experienced "a noticeable relaxation of the pressure and distension within an hour and no recurrence of the problem thereafter."[8]

The appearance of this article was the first major public introduction of acupuncture to the Western world. The following year, the National Acupuncture Association, which helped provide training in acupuncture to Western doctors, was founded in the US. Later that year, Nixon made his tour of China; afterward, Major General Walter R. Tkach, Nixon's personal physician, joining Reston's media crusade, wrote an article for *Reader's Digest* called "I Watched Acupuncture Work." He reported on the use of acupuncture as an anesthetic during surgeries in China. Other American doctors soon visited China and made similar claims, including President Eisenhower's former physician, who described seeing a patient given nothing but acupuncture as an anesthetic during a complicated brain operation. Subsequently, there was a surge of public interest in America, and the news caught the eye of the medical establishment as well. Later in 1973, the IRS began allowing acupuncture to be deducted as a legitimate medical expense. Interest in complementary healing modalities grew steadily enough after that for the US Congress to create, in 1992, the Office of Alternative Medicine. In 1998, the National Institutes of Health (NIH) created the National Center for Complementary and Alternative Medicine—renamed in 2014 as the National Center for Complementary and Integrative Health[9]—a government agency meant to define the usefulness and safety of medical and health care not generally considered part of conventional medicine in the context of rigorous science. (Recent studies have included research on the use of music therapy to relieve stress; an exploration of the way people perceive prospective and actual pain and how this affects the autonomic nervous system; and, my personal favorite, how a cup of coffee can potentially reduce acupuncture's effect on pain.[10])

Today more than three million Americans have tried acupuncture, and most major hospitals have integrated the treatment in some form, as we did at Lutheran. Medical centers such as the Cleveland Clinic have brought Chinese herbs into their repertoire. (At my clinic, too, we prescribe herbs and use moxa or moxibustion—the same *ai ye*, the "broken cheap cigar" Reston mentioned in his article.) Additionally, the National Institutes of Health now recommends that a working knowledge of acupuncture be taught in medical schools.[11]

Recently, too, there has been a proliferation of studies that show acupuncture has measurable physiological effects, diminishing the idea that once dominated the medical world that acupuncture was simply a "theatrical placebo,"[12] as one journal put it. Doppler ultrasound has been used to show that acupuncture increases blood flow and circulation,[13] and MRI readings demonstrate that acupuncture can prompt observable changes in the brain. Wide-ranging research suggests that acupuncture can do everything from improve sleep[14] to increase blood flow in the umbilical cord of pregnant women to easing mental health struggles. (One 2013 study published in the *Journal of Alternative and Complementary Medicine* found that electroacupuncture—a form of acupuncture in which a mild electric current is transmitted through the needles—was as effective as Prozac in reducing symptoms of depression.[15])

And yet we are still left without a complete picture of *why* acupuncture works. Science—with its eternal desire for a precise answer—has made many efforts to come up with a sound reason. As a result, various theories have been presented over the decades.

One of the first explanations put forth is known as the endorphin theory. American researchers, intrigued by acupuncture as a powerful anesthetic (based on the reports of Nixon's doctor and others) but unable to accept the TCM explanation of energetic "channels" of the body, proposed that the insertion of needles released a flood of endorphins, the body's natural painkillers. Research does, in fact, show that administering acupuncture leads to an endorphin release in humans as well as in some animals[16]—which may account for the contented, floaty feeling people often report after treatment—but there is doubt as to whether these endorphins are directly responsible for the reported reduction in pain.[17] In one study,[18] for instance, researchers used acupuncture for pain relief during dental surgery. Once the patients had experienced measurable relief from the acupuncture, they were then given an opiate antagonist, Naloxone. This drug is often given to people who have overdosed on narcotics, because it blocks their effects. And it works equally well to block the effects of endogenous opioids, the innate pain-relieving system that includes endorphins. The idea being: if the presence of endorphins explains acupuncture's pain-relieving effects, the patients' suffering would increase once they were given Naloxone. And yet this didn't happen in most studies—though some did show a moderate effect. This made clear that an increase in the body's natural painkiller, although helpful, does not explain how acupuncture would give sufficient pain relief to anesthetize patients during surgery.

The endorphin idea was soon merged with another theory adapted from an already well-established notion in Western medicine called the "gate-control theory of pain." The "gate" in the name refers to the spinal cord, which acts as a filter for the nervous system, controlling which signals should be allowed up to the brain. Constant stimulation will eventually close the gate; lack of stimulation will leave the gate open so that your brain can register a new sensation. When this theory is applied to acupuncture, the idea is that the needles, offering stimulation, close the gate, shutting down pain in the body, and possibly also triggering a change in the brain physiology that would release endorphins or neurotransmitters that decrease the sensation of pain.[19]

Later, another hypothesis suggested that the tiny—and, I should add, painless—wounds the needles cause in a person's body ramp up the immune system, jump-starting the healing process. Specifically, the prick of the needle sends a message to the body that causes inflammatory proteins and other infection-fighting, would-be healing chemicals to flood the site of the injury, revving the immune system to deal with any bigger problems as well.[20]

Each of these theories offers a distinct explanation for how acupuncture affects the body—and every one is right, albeit incomplete. By that I mean that acupuncture isn't just one kind of intervention. As an acupuncturist, I use the needles in different ways in response to the particular needs of each patient. If someone has sciatica, I needle along the course of the sciatic nerve, interrupting its signal—which could be called the gate theory—but I might also choose to place the needles directly into a muscle spasm to release the knots, which is more of a mechanical intervention similar in outcome to massage. I will also often treat acupuncture points throughout the body that prompt a release of a patient's endorphins with a view toward helping them relax. (Patients sometimes ask me, "What do you put in the needles?" They grow so serene during sessions, they assume I've coated my needles in some sort of sedative. I explain that they are experiencing a natural chemical reaction, one that can make you feel as if you've taken a Valium—without actually taking a Valium.)

Since America's introduction to acupuncture came through the lens of pain relief, most of the hypothesizing about how it worked focused on its analgesic benefits. But acupuncture's effects on the body are more complex and sophisticated than is commonly understood. I, myself, primarily practice internal medicine—such as working to improve the condition of a specific organ or helping women to get pregnant by balancing reproductive hormones. From my perspective, then, these theories only tell part of the story. They don't, after all, answer some of the more profound and mysterious questions about acupuncture's potency. Why did the cervixes of the women in labor at Lutheran dilate more quickly with acupuncture? How does needling a point on the leg or the foot cause a reaction in the uterus, an organ that, by all medical logic, is not at all related to those parts of the body? Why is it that if you perform acupuncture on the scalp of stroke patients at a particular point of the brain, as I learned to do from a Chinese practitioner, they gain mobility of their previously paralyzed left arms?[21]

As such, I went in search of a theory that would encompass all of acupuncture's powers—from pain relief to fertility treatment to spectacular recovery. I had a feeling that the research would hint at the importance of the needle grab.

For this, I had to go back to the beginning. I had to look at the development of the embryo and how it organizes itself in terms of setting up a mode of communication throughout the body.

Several years ago, at an acupuncture conference in Vancouver,

I met a British surgeon and emergency medical specialist named Dan Keown. He was at this conference because he also happens to be a certified acupuncturist. At the time, Keown had caused a stir in Chinese medical circles because he'd recently published a book that asked a simple yet disarming question (and one that he was uniquely suited to answer): What could Western doctors learn by studying Eastern medicine?

In his book, *The Spark in the Machine: How the Science of Acupuncture Explains the Mysteries of Western Medicine*,[22] Keown makes a strong argument—based in large part on the research of Charles Shang, a professor and researcher at Baylor College of Medicine—that the human embryo develops nodes that function as organizing centers, dictating how our bodies take shape as well as creating an electrical network that corresponds with the acupuncture points and channels of Chinese medicine.

As Keown describes it, at no time is an organism's ability to systematize more impressive than during embryogenesis. "The level of [organization] required to make a human baby is quite simply staggering," he writes. "In nine months, a single cell will multiply until it is 10,000,000,000,000 cells. This alone is quite a feat, but while it does this it will [organize] itself into everything that we take for granted in good health."[23]

As most communication in the body is mediated by either the nervous system or through the blood, common sense would have us believe these same systems are at work during embryogenesis. And yet, upon closer study, this seems unlikely. By the fourth week of pregnancy, the embryo is just a quarter inch long, smaller than a grain of rice. The nervous system and blood vessels have begun to form but they are too poorly developed to act as communication channels. Still, somehow each cell—and there are over twenty thousand of them at this point—knows exactly what to do.

The biological process that causes an organism to develop its shape is known as morphogenesis (from the Greek *morphê*, literally meaning "beginning of the shape"). In the embryo, this is accomplished by morphogens, powerful growth factors specific to embryonic cells. Morphogens do not need to travel through the blood to work. Instead they diffuse through the spaces between cells. If a certain type of morphogen reaches a specific level of concentration, then it prompts the embryo to grow a new limb, organ, or other structure, by activating the genes involved in that process. The term "morphogens" was coined, remarkably, by renowned World War II Nazi code-breaker Alan Turing in his 1952 paper, "The Chemical Basis for Morphogenesis,[24] in which he describes a chemical and mathematical model to explain how an embryo grows.

In systems theory, many components interact with one another, using organizational centers, where lines of communication intersect and are disseminated efficiently, creating a chain of command. This, Turing proposed, is also the method by which an embryo directs its growth. The organizational centers, or nodes, of our bodies are collections of specialized cells. Unlike the cells around them, however, they don't move, grow, or differentiate. Instead they regulate and control the cells around them, giving orders to grow an arm or a kidney or the lens of an eye.

The existence of such nodes was discovered, albeit in amphibians, in the 1930s, when German embryologist Hans Spemann identified the areas of embryos that direct the development of

groups of cells into particular tissues and organs and limbs. Spemann was even able to transplant nodes into a second embryo in
his experiments and, in so doing, also transplanted their control
of growth and development. In effect, Spemann was able to bring
Salvador Dalí–like creatures to life by manipulating the organizing centers to build a salamander with two heads and frogs with
eyelids all over their bodies. (Incidentally, Spemann, in 1928,
was the first to perform somatic cell nuclear transfer—creating a
viable embryo from a body cell and an egg cell—setting an early
precedent for cloning.) Seven years later, in 1935, he was awarded
the Nobel Prize in Physiology for Medicine "for the discovery of
the organizer effect in embryologic development."

These organizing centers, or nodes, Keown points out, are
consistently located at major acupuncture points. And they form
a network that looks remarkably like the acupuncture channel
map of traditional Chinese medicine. (The acupuncture points
and channels have been consistently identified in research: a
2014 study,[25] published in the *Journal of Electron Spectroscopy and
Related Phenomena*, used CT scan imaging, with synchrotron
radiation [offering a more sophisticated readout], of acupuncture
points and nonacupuncture points. It showed that the acupuncture points had a greater number of small blood vessels that curl
inward or bifurcate around large, thicker blood vessels. Additionally, these points and channels have been identified in other
experiments using MRIs,[26] infrared imaging, LCD thermal photography,[27] and ultrasound.[28])

Are the acupuncture points then the remains of early embryological organizing centers? Harvard graduate and assistant
professor of medicine at Baylor Charles Shang—whose research

Keown expands upon in his book[29]—has investigated this in a series[30] of papers published starting in 2001.[31] In these, Shang introduced his Growth Control Theory of Acupuncture, offering a bioenergetic illustration of the acupuncture map of the body. Over the course of his work, Shang has also shown that the specialized cells that form our nodes continue to have a regulatory function throughout our lives. "Once humans are mature they need to maintain control rather than install it," Keown writes, meaning that the body's organizing system—and the electrical energy, what Chinese medicine would call qi, that runs through it—is at its most powerful when we are young and then ages along with us, not disappearing but shifting in its function.

If nodes translate into the acupuncture points, then what is the biological explanation for the channels—or pathways—along which our electrical energy travels? As an embryo grows ever more complex, it divides into compartments, clearly delineating one part of the body from the other. These compartments are enclosed with a specialized connective tissue, primarily made up of collagen, known as "fascia."

Fascia is found everywhere in our bodies. It underpins our skin; it also attaches, stabilizes, encloses, and separates muscles and other internal organs. There are three forms of it—superficial, deep (which is the connective tissue affected by acupuncture), and visceral; it is intimately involved with nourishing all cells of the body, including those of disease. It is also extremely strong, "so strong," as Keown points out, "that in the days of Björn Borg and John McEnroe, professional players' tennis strings were made from the fascia from the gut of a cow."[32] Fascia is impenetrable to almost all biological substances; it is so impassable that it becomes a kind of slide, or slippery pathway, for a number of things in our bodies: water, air, blood, and even electricity. In fact, not only is fascia an electrical conductor and resistor, capable of transmitting electrical signals throughout the body, but it can also, amazingly, generate its own electricity.[33]

Fascia, then, it is theorized, is the conduit for electrical energy, or qi, as it travels throughout our bodies. "These pathways of fascia have been detailed beautifully by anatomists," Keown points out, "only they were not describing the fascia but the tissues that they enclosed."[34] It is even a principle of surgery to cut along the fascial planes—conscious always not to cut into the fascia unless absolutely necessary as it leads to an increased risk of adhesions, essentially cutting across the body's system of organization—without realizing that these pathways are not simply there to make their incisions easier. "When the West talks of fascial planes, the East talks of acupuncture channels," Keown writes. "There is no contraindication in these two views; it is just a question of interpretation. The West may still have no comparable force to [qi], but that is only because it has not attempted to explain the holistic power behind embryological self-organization."[35]

(Incidentally, fascia also plays a key role in demystifying an anomaly that sometimes occurs in acupuncture research. In some studies, researchers use "sham acupuncture"—which can mean administering needles at non–acupuncture points or using retractable needles that do not penetrate the skin—to measure its effects against "real" acupuncture. In some of these studies, legitimate acupuncture only works slightly better than its sham counterpart, leading some researchers to conclude that acupuncture, in general, is nothing more than a placebo. However, given the conductive nature of fascia, needling anywhere along a fascial plane should have some conductive effect, if not as strong as when treating at the accurate points. As for the needles that don't penetrate the skin, acupressure or shallow needling can create a small oscillation that stimulates the electrical activity enough to mildly activate the acupuncture points.[36])

Western medicine has, however, begun to investigate—and accept—the idea that bioelectric signals are necessary for body formation. In 2011, a pair of Tufts biologists released research, accompanied by a video[37] (now living on in Google infamy as "Electric Frog Face"), reporting their discovery that bioelectric signals cause groups of cells to form the patterns to create the head and facial formation of a frog, and they had captured the process in a time-lapse film.

"Our research shows that the electrical state of a cell is fundamental to development. Bioelectrical signaling appears to regulate a sequence of events, not just one," said Laura Vandenberg, the first author on the paper published in *Developmental Dynamics*. "Developmental biologists are used to thinking of sequences in which a gene produces a protein product that in turn ultimately leads to development of an eye or a mouth. But our work suggests that something else—a bioelectrical signal—is required before that can happen."[38]

The Tufts team also found that disrupting bioelectric signaling correlated with craniofacial abnormalities. Some embryos grew two brains rather than one; others had thickened optic nerves or lacked normal nasal or jaw development.

"These findings suggest that what we thought about how cells know what to make is incomplete," concluded Vandenberg, "and this is a way to sort of finish that story—or take a new road for that story." Or even to revisit research from the past: recall Robert O. Becker's work with amputated salamanders (discussed in Chapter 2) and his discovery that there was a shift in electric charge at the stump—suggesting energetic potential—as the limb began to grow back again.

"Electric Frog Face" not only builds on Becker's work, it also affirms the work of Keown and Shang, both of whom have put forth that there is a specific type of electrical signal—to their minds, qi—that is directing the pattern of cells.

Chinese medicine, however, puts an emphasis on the changing nature of qi, at once a material substance and an ethereal force that integrates mind, body, and spirit. Everything in the universe, from our bodies to the stars, is the result of a continuous cycle, the coming together and then dispersal of qi. "If we define qi as an organizational energy, then that works in the cosmos. There is order there as well," as Keown described it when we spoke,[39] "[which] is the high aim of physics—the holy grail of physics— the idea that there is one force that explains everything." Our personal energy field, our qi, is not only the body's intelligence and organizing system, but also a microcosm of the biggest field of all, the field from which life itself emerges, the Tao.

I never understood this better than when, still in school in San Diego, I bumped into one of my teachers, Z'ev Rosenberg, when I was taking a walk on the beach. He was standing at the edge of the ocean staring out into the water. In Chinese medicine, our initial clues for diagnosis come from taking the pulse, which offers varying speeds and depths for different organs. When I asked Z'ev what he was doing, he said he was practicing his pulse diagnosis. "The ripples on the shore are the result of the bigger waves farther out, so they reflect them," he told me. Similarly, the wrist's pulse carries an energetic vibration from deep inside the body. The ancient Chinese relied on this information because they didn't have diagnostic tools like we do today, yet the intricate system of pulse diagnosis works just as well now as it did thousands of years ago. There is a reason that acupuncture has stood the test of time. At its most elemental, it is positing that we are capable of healing in response to a charge, a surge of new information, just as the universe, or the Tao, is constantly changing in response to information from us.

YOU THE HEALER

Acupressure

Given the embryological significance of the acupuncture points, it's time to learn about some of the most important ones in the body. You can massage these points, in a technique known as acupressure, which will generate and transmit energy through the body. A trained acupuncturist would use these points as part of a complete treatment, using a variety of locations to address the patient's whole symptom pattern. For our purposes, though, we're going to use them to address a specific region of the body.

LARGE INTESTINE 4

If you look at the back of your hand and press your thumb of that same hand into the side of your hand, you'll notice that a crease is made. At the end of that crease is a bulge. Press your opposite thumb into the muscle at the highest point of the bulge. Press toward the hand. Roll around until you find a sensitive area. Hold this, with steady pressure, for a few minutes or until the sensitivity decreases.

You can use this point for any problems in the head and neck, including facial pain, toothache, headache, or neck and shoulder tension.

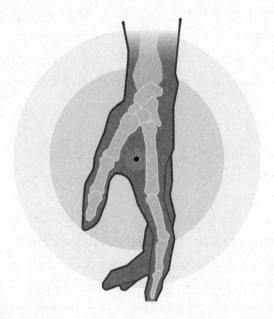

STOMACH 36
Slide your hand down from the outside of your kneecap along the outer boundary of your shinbone and you will find a little hollow about four finger widths down from the bottom of your kneecap. Massage this area, with steady pressure, for a few minutes or until the sensitivity decreases.

The Chinese name for this point is Zu San Li, which is often translated as "three-leg-mile." In ancient times, Chinese soldiers were encouraged to rub this point to help them march an extra three miles. You can use it to generate energy, too, as well as for digestive problems.

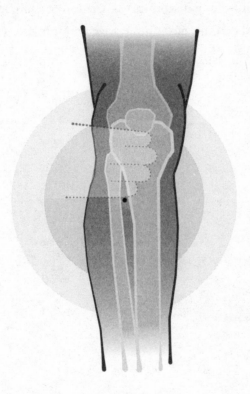

SPLEEN 6

Reach down to your inner ankle and find the bone that sticks out (it's called the medial malleolus). Slide your finger three fingers' breadth up from the center of the medial malleolus (in the illustration, the bottom fourth finger is resting on the medial malleolus) and find an area that feels like a hollow or sensitive spot. Massage this area, with steady pressure, for a few minutes or until the sensitivity decreases.

This is the acupuncture point I was using in the hospital to relieve labor pain. Because of its effect on the uterus, it shouldn't be used in pregnancy except during labor. If you're not pregnant, you can use it for any discomfort in the lower abdomen, including menstrual cramps, gas, or digestive cramping.

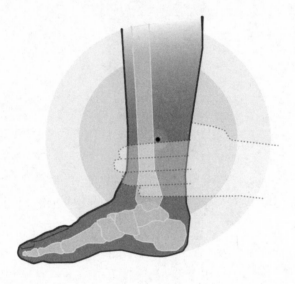

6

HANDS-ON ACTIVITIES

In 2012, as Yinova, my clinical practice, was expanding, I hired a naturopath named Carla Kreft to work with our patients. Naturopathic doctors are physicians who are educated in the same basic sciences as medical doctors and use the same standard Western medical diagnoses, but they take a holistic approach, encouraging patients to consider the underlying causes for their illnesses, and they primarily treat with natural remedies. The first thing I'd ever heard about Carla—aside from the fact that the well-respected head of her naturopathic school told me that she was the brightest student he'd ever taught—was that she comes from a long line of Peruvian healers and mystics and that witnesses once saw her thrown across the room by an evil spirit. At the very least, I thought, I had to meet this woman.

Carla not only enriched my practice, but also transformed the way in which I saw myself as a practitioner. Her work ethos gracefully aligned with mine—she is a rigorous naturopath with a biomedical slant as well as a profound healer—but she also possessed a clarity of purpose that I wasn't always able to access myself. In other words, she had a bracing, no-bullshit attitude that I adored.

One day early on in her time at Yinova, after she'd observed me administer acupuncture to a patient, she lingered by the door of the treatment room. She had a great look: a Queens mom with a shamanic edge. On that day her black hair was pulled back into a loose bun, a dusting of gray throughout, and her playful, knowing brown eyes told me she had something to tell me. So I gestured toward her, as if to say, *Let's hear it.*

She smiled and said, "You know you don't need the needles anymore, right?" Yes, actually, I did know, and had known for a while, though I'd resisted admitting it even to myself. But Carla was right: the needles were no longer essential to the work I was doing.

And yet I didn't want to let them go. I had come to rely on the needles, and on acupuncture as a whole. For one, I felt being a licensed professional had given me a respected place in the medical community. I was proud to practice Chinese medicine. I'd worked hard to become licensed as an acupuncturist—it had taken rigor and discipline to pass my medical boards. And, once I became a practitioner, I found that the foundations of Chinese medicine provided the structure I needed to manage my patients' cases in a way that helped them. This not only kept me humble—I knew I was standing on the shoulders of giants—but it also kept me honest. It was crucial to me to offer a service I knew was beneficial.

I worried then about stepping away from a legitimate field of energy work, with high educational and ethical standards,[1] and wandering into a world that was largely unregulated. It felt to me a bit like venturing into the Wild West. There are many energy workers who are talented and effective—I'd already met a good number of them in my effort to understand how energy medicine works—but scattered among them are also the unscrupulous, the snake oil salesmen and would-be gurus. These people gravitate to the fringes of alternative medicine, where training is optional and oversight is negligible. Over the years, I'd had my fair share of encounters with them as well as witnessed some of my patients be taken in by them.

I also felt safely hemmed in by acupuncture on a personal level. For as long as I'd had an intuitive sense of my ability to heal, I'd had a conjoined instinct that it was just plain weird. I fought this, as I knew logically it was a pointless inhibition, but I couldn't stop myself from feeling a deep sense of refusal when I considered shifting my role to "energy healer." (Though acupuncture is also a type of energy work—meaning that technically I was already an energy healer—this new realm of energy medicine, using only my hands as a conduit, felt vastly different.) When I'd worked with Andrew, my patient who'd had prostate cancer, twelve years earlier, I had used hands-on healing—and despite the fact that I could sense a healing force run through me in our sessions, I'd felt a bit unstable without the needles to ground me as a practitioner. Since then, I'd had it both ways. I had the security of the needles and the solid history of acupuncture backing me as well as the space to explore connecting to a larger energy source when it felt right.

At the time, I tried, with less fluency and intelligibility, as stated above, to explain this to Carla. But she wasn't having it. "You have more power than you understand," she urged. "I can see you're only using a fraction of your skills because you're scared."

And so I asked her to show me how she heals people with her own kind of energy healing. By this time, I'd already met Bill Bengston, so I knew his technique, and, of course, I was well versed in my own more intuitive method. But I was especially curious to learn from Carla because her practice developed from a combination of lessons learned from the spiritual adepts of her Peruvian family and an unusual gnostic Egyptian healing tradition. Between the two, she had learned to see, and use, spirit guides to tap into the body's chakras for information and to access otherworldly dimensions. ("I can describe in detail the carpet on the staircase of your childhood home," she said by way of an example of how she might tap into a seemingly inaccessible realm.)

Though Carla herself, out of respect for tribal traditions, does not refer to herself as a shaman, much of what she practices overlaps with this practice. Shamanism in its primitive form—stripping back the egregious layers of new age interpretations that we, in the West, have projected onto it in recent history—embodies the spiritual wisdom of a variety of indigenous tribes. The term "shamanism" was, in fact, first offered by Western anthropologists when observing the ancient religion of the Turks and Mongols as well as neighboring tribes in Siberia, China, and northernmost Eurasia. Over time, Western anthropologists began to use the term in a broad sense, encompassing unrelated rituals found within religions of other parts of Asia, Africa, Australasia, and some parts of the Americas. More recently, shamanism has been appropriated by pop healing culture, with practitioners in large cities, such as Manhattan, Los Angeles, and Sydney, offering a conflation of energy healing, meditation, astrological guidance, and—I kid you not—private jet sessions.

At base, however, shamanism describes the ability of a person to serve as an intermediary, or messenger, between the spirit world and the human world. Typically, a shaman can enter a trance state—or, as the Romanian historian Mircea Eliade put it, a "religious ecstasy"[2]—in order to offer guidance and healing. Carla describes herself, in particular, and shamans, in general, as "someone who has a very strong connection to nature and understands the world through these natural forces."[3] The practice of shamanism, however, varies geographically. Carla, whose family is from a small jungle village near Iquitos, the largest city in the Peruvian Amazon, explained that even within Peruvian shamanism, there is a marked difference between those who practice in the jungle and those who practice in the mountains. "It's a cosmological difference," she says. "In the mountains, they have a different vocabulary; the ceremonies are different; the music is different; the diet is different; the entire process is different because of the region."[4]

Iquitos is also a popular destination for "ayahuasca tourism," where Westerners gather to take the hallucinogenic made from roots and vines specific to the region. Although some groups have a religious exemption, for the most part it is illegal to distribute ayahuasca in the United States. Such is its popularity, however, that many people, myself included, have tried it, often traveling abroad to do so. Ayahuasca is only one of the thousands of herbal remedies that shamans use, and Carla believes that it should be treated with respect and not taken casually. As she explained, "Ayahuasca requires a commitment to a specific lifestyle; the indigenous people use rituals to prepare themselves to take it."[5] Their preparation may include periods of sexual celibacy, strict diets, and special trials—such as spending three days alone in the jungle in order to face their fears. The preparation is designed to reduce the participants' cravings and lust for earthly pleasures such as sex or food as well as to help them face their own demons. With this kind of preparation, the participant can interpret the ayahuasca trip with more clarity and less fear and the result can be a profoundly spiritual experience.[6]

Interestingly, like me, Carla also had a fairly traumatic childhood—her father struggled with alcoholism, making her feel "there were dangers at home"—and describes a similar sense of always being on high alert as a consequence. "I never knew what was coming next," she confides. "As a result, I learned to read people."[7]

So I felt I was in both capable and compassionate hands when I entered my own treatment room one afternoon and lay down on the table so Carla could treat me. Initially, she talked me through similar exercises to the ones I've offered in this book: I visualized a grounding cord, like an anchor, rooting me to the earth and then imagined light pouring through me. In this instance, though, I was learning, by observing Carla, how to instruct the patient to do this as well. Carla stood behind my head, narrating along the way what she was visualizing—which, at that point, was my spiritual energy as a flooding stream of light. She guided this stream of light through my crown chakra and into my body. I felt euphoric and light when she did this, like a barely tethered balloon that could take off at any moment. Then she walked around to the other end of the table, to my feet, and visualized bringing up the earth's energy, which immediately grounded the airy feeling I had just felt and made me feel peaceful. She pulled that through my feet into my body to meet the light. I shut my eyes and began to see vivid colors. I was conscious of Carla waving her arms above me and movement in my body as it responded.

Her shamanistic training gives Carla access to the energy that runs between us, which she sees as a web of lines that connect as they cross one another. It also means that, like Kiran, she can see areas of stuck energy. This sense of connection is expressed in Chinese medicine too. Chinese philosophers say we are a microcosm of the greater energy field, individual representations of the Tao; the shamans say we are connected to a spiritual realm we cannot see but we can feel. This notion is echoed in the laws of physics, which assert that we are energy condensed into physical form—the same energy that exists at large in the universe.

I had already arrived at parts of Carla's ritual naturally—I had been, for instance, imagining filling my patients with light during treatments for some time—but I hadn't been asking my patients to visualize as well during treatments. Given my ambivalence about announcing my healing strengths, I hadn't allowed for a sense of structure about it. Carla helped me to accept—and discipline—my natural aptitude for energy healing.

She also taught me, in that session, about chakras. I'd contemplated chakras before, of course—particularly when I'd worked in hospice and could feel the energy of a dying patient leaving through the crown chakra—but I hadn't yet brought them into my practice as a source of healing. Though chakras are considered an Indian concept ("chakra" is a Sanskrit word)—and correlate to acupuncture in that they are located at major acupuncture points in the middle of the body—Carla had picked up on them as powerful energy centers and had incorporated them into her work. In general, Carla, building on the foundation of her cultural inheritance, draws from the various parts of her eclectic training to create a healing treatment all her own.

"When I am healing, in some people, I sense something more physical; it's deeper and within the boundary of their body. With others, I feel something outside of the body but within their energetic field," Carla told me that day. "Either way, I am always able to feel their chakras. The chakras are on the border of the physical and the nonphysical."[8] Carla was able to perceive not only these whirling energy centers, but also the entire energy field around the body, sometimes called the aura (and also referred to as "the corona discharge" by Kirlian, the photographer from Chapter 2). The chakras and the body's energy field work together as an integrated system—the chakras being the points at which information enters and leaves the body.

There are seven main chakras, or "wheels," as translated from the Sanskrit. Each one, it is believed, plays a specific role in keeping a person in balance. The first one, for example, is the root chakra (Muladhara), which is meant to help with a person's daily survival or, as Carla describes it, a person's sense of "belonging to this world; the very basic question: 'Do I have a right to be here?'" (See the meditation at the end of this chapter for an explanation of all the chakras.)

"I personally work with people almost as if it is a checkup," Carla explained. "I go one by one, to each chakra, and project some energy from my hand through the front [of a person's body] and feel how it comes out the back. If the chakra is healthy, if the size is appropriate, the movement is easy, I can feel the energy I project from the front come out the back. If, on the other hand, there is a problem, it can be very weak or slow moving, similar to a pulse. Sometimes, if someone is very blocked, I project energy from the front and it just kind of disappears into nowhere." It is also possible to have too much activity—"the equivalent of a scattered pulse";[9] these people are spilling out energy, according to Carla, and need it brought back within their control. She taught me how to feel the chakras; each one is shaped like a cone and is positioned within as if it were pointed toward the front of a person's body, broadening out toward the back. If the person is healthy, the chakra rotates.

Carla also talked of reaching a meditative, almost hypnotic state in her more intensive sessions, moving outward toward other realms, until finally she reached a place where there are no laws of time and space. "If I wanted to I could touch someone in my family's energy field in Peru right now," she said. "It's almost like a highway—there are lines, or frequencies, that crisscross always. The longer you can stay there, the more this dimension opens itself up to you."[10]

Carla possesses an alluring nonchalance, and a trustworthiness, that I wish I could capture on the page in a more visceral way. Some of these ideas are hard to contemplate; they're too far out of the realm of our everyday considerations. There is a way that Carla communicates, not only without self-consciousness but also with such a bright and pioneering quality, you just fall into line with her. Carla explained that reaching the realm she spoke of—without time or space—is not unlike glimpsing enlightenment or the Tao. "We think of enlightenment as the thing we need to work so hard to arrive at, but every tradition will tell you it is within you," she reminded me. "They are not exaggerating. And they are not saying, 'It is within you in a deep, dark cavern that you can never find.' It's not out of reach . . . but I can only manage to stay in this state for a few minutes at a time. In those minutes, though, I am not yearning for anything. It feels like physical and emotional contentment, which permits a lightness toward life that comes from knowing with 100 percent surety that there is a calm source that exists parallel with our daily life in the here and now. It's only a matter of willingly shifting your perspective. I experience this state as being present in the spaces between our cells. It is a hyperawareness of being the consciousness that is the observer of life, and in that state you are released from the weight of striving. This is the state I endeavor to enter at some point during a healing session."[11]

I thought of Kiran Trace—who so abruptly lost her sense of identity and began to "see where formlessness, or space, encodes to form"[12]—and of Bill Bengston, who had described feeling "pervaded with peace and well-being. My mind emptied of thought"[13] while healing the mice in the lab. I wondered if all of us trying to narrate these experiences were reaching the same conclusion—or realm—and were just feeling about for the right way to describe it.

After that lesson—and some more coaxing from Carla—I began to practice energy healing more openly with some of my longtime acupuncture patients. I would explain to them that acupuncture is a form of energy medicine and ask if they were comfortable with me bringing energy healing to the fore in our sessions. It was a pronounced shift for me—openly announcing that I wanted to include this as a part of my treatments—and it was useful. As I became more accustomed to it, and less self-conscious about it, I was able to tap into it with more command.

And I learned an enormous amount. I found that if I concentrated on opening my crown chakra, as I'd done with Carla, and let the energy permeate me, I felt the same back-straightening tingling down my spine that I'd felt with Andrew and now my right hand instinctually went up into the air while my left hand, facing down toward my patients' bodies, grew warmer. I was grateful that most of my patients fell asleep, or at least closed their eyes, while I worked on them, as I still felt a bit self-conscious about letting loose in this way. One of my patients who'd stayed awake, however, and observed the whole ritual, said I looked like an Egyptian hieroglyph. But, regardless of whether they saw me in Egyptian hieroglyph mode or not, most of them responded enthusiastically to these treatments: they were not only healing physically but they came out with a sense of emotional balance as well.

The energy work, in addition to the acupuncture, seemed to speed up healing. It seemed particularly good for unraveling complex, chronic cases, as if the information that was coming through me was allowing the body to reorganize. Patients also reported feeling less depressed or anxious; they told me they were sleeping better. One patient who'd seen me for years as an acupuncturist had, initially, when I'd first started introducing more energy work, laughed about this strange new turn I'd taken. But then he'd also always been quite healthy, seeing me for maintenance or "tune-ups" more than anything else—until, that is, he broke both his legs in a skiing accident. When I treated him after that, I hovered my hand above the breaks, and his legs literally began to shake and his toes curled involuntarily. Both of us were a bit taken aback by the strength of the connection—I was, it seemed, responding more vigorously because of his greater need. He was, after that, able to refer to me as his "energy healer"— with an almost straight face.

With acupuncture, I felt as if I were affecting the patients' personal energy fields, whereas when I relinquished the needles, I felt as if I were directing energy from the larger field, from Tao, or source, to the patient. Both were effective—and, therefore, satisfying to me as a practitioner—but I did feel that I had entered a larger arena, so to speak, when I was trying out energy healing with just my hands. As I began to deepen my work, I, too, experienced periods of time when I was able to observe my physical body from outside and experience my consciousness as separate. At these times I would feel connected to a vast source of intelligence; I could feel it run through me and connect me to a realm where I did feel we really were all one. At these times, I understood with a depth and certainty I hadn't reached before that my body, a temporary expression of physicality, was also a way in which source could make itself known.

At about the same time that this shift was occurring in my energy work practice, I got a call from a young woman in London who announced that she was the assistant to a Middle Eastern prince, who from here on out I will simply call "the prince." The prince had heard of a woman in New York with "magnetic hands" and had asked his assistant to find her. I wasn't even sure I was the person he was looking for, but after a recommendation from the prince's massage therapist (someone I'd met before profession-ally), her search had landed with me. The young woman asked if I would be willing to come work with the prince for three weeks on his yacht that summer. The prince, she said, didn't like nee-dles so didn't want acupuncture. He wanted an energy healer.

In the weeks approaching my departure, the plans kept shift-ing, as the yacht charted its course along the Mediterranean. First I was to meet them in Santorini, then Sardinia, and finally, doubling back to Greece, in Athens. I was sent a plane ticket, told to go to a particular hotel and then await further instructions. Once there, I was told a car would pick me up in the morning and drive me to the coast, where I'd be met by a tender to ferry me to the boat. I was starting to feel as if I'd been cast as an extra in *Ocean's Eleven*.

Eventually, however, I arrived at the superyacht—it was the size of a cruise ship; I could hardly believe it was all in service of one person—with my suitcase in one hand and acupuncture equipment in the other (this I'd brought as a backup, in case all else failed with my energy healing). I settled into my room with its private bath that faced a porthole offering an alluring glimpse of the Greek coastline. I met the prince briefly that night—we had a polite exchange, though I said very little (as his staff had advised me to do earlier in the afternoon). There was such a sense of formal expectation I had to fight the instinct to curtsy. It was a surreal experience, for all the obvious reasons, but also because I was so used to building a rapport with my patients. Here, with the prince, though, there was a cool distance, and protocol, it seemed, would make it impossible to come any closer.

The next morning the captain of the ship, a fellow Brit, came to me and said, "Dr. Jill, His Highness has asked if we can anchor off the temple in Delphi this afternoon so that you can gather energy from it together during his treatment." This was, hands down, one of the strangest conversations to occur between two British people without one of us cracking a smile—still, we forged ahead. "He'd like you on deck two hours before the treatment to meditate in preparation," the captain continued. "We'll arrange a space for you on His Highness's private sundeck." I agreed and went back to my room to Google "Delphi."

Delphi, as I learned from my Internet search belowdecks, was considered the center, or "navel," of the earth by the ancient Greeks and was known for its oracle, the high priestess of the Temple of Apollo, sometimes referred to as Pythia, who was consulted about important decisions throughout the classical world. Legend has it that when Apollo slayed a python, its body fell into a fissure in the earth, where fumes arose from its decomposing body. The oracle, perched above the crack in the earth, would become intoxicated by the vapors and fall into a trance. Apollo would then possess her spirit and, in this state, she would prophesy.

I went to the sundeck to meditate, seeking my inner Pythia and feeling thoroughly intimidated. As I stood there, though, practicing the exercises I'd learned with Carla, putting my anchor down and flooding myself with my own healing light, I began to relax. After a time, I felt a familiar whir of energy, that pleasant effervescent feeling I'd become accustomed to experiencing before treatments. I was elated and relieved that the energy I had felt in my clinic was coming through, that I had something real to offer the prince. Everything took on a dreamlike quality. His Highness came at the appointed time, thanked me in advance, and took his place on the massage table set up by the pool. I grounded him and filled him with his own light before checking and opening his chakras. The prince went to sleep. I continued to work and allowed my body to be a conduit. As I worked I could sense the movement of his chakras, and I found I could see areas of blockage that showed up as opaque areas above his body—with a particular feeling of burden around his shoulders—and I tried to push this energy down through his grounding cord (I had asked him to imagine having one). At the end of our session, the prince woke up and remarked that he felt lighter. And then went off to Jet Ski.

The conditions of my stay on the yacht—that I should spend the day getting ready to treat the prince by meditating, doing yoga, eating well—would have been ideal at any point in my life but, in particular, at this time, it helped to bolster my confidence and accelerate my skills as a healer. And, with so much time devoted to my practice, some bold things did happen. Once, for example, as I was working with the prince, while in the dreamy state I was by then regularly experiencing, I suddenly saw a hand—not my own—stroke his head. It was a strikingly clear image: the elegant, albeit disembodied, hand of a woman. After that treatment, the prince commented, "It's an amazing skill that you have. You're lucky to have this talent." I was too conscious of our yacht decorum to ask him anything more, but I do still wonder what he was thinking or dreaming about as I was practicing that day.

I came home unambiguously convinced of my ability to use energy to heal. And yet I also knew that I would never give up the needles. There was no need: the two practices were not mutually exclusive. Given my newfound certainty about my abilities, however, I decided to concentrate on my shamanic exploration.

I recalled a pilgrimage I'd made to a woman I'll call Master Yang, a qigong practitioner whom I'd heard about from a colleague; she purported to be able to materialize herbs in her hands. Qigong is a holistic system relying on movement, breathing, meditation, and herbs to cultivate health and spirituality. It has roots in Chinese medicine, philosophy, and martial arts; its primary goal, not unlike acupuncture, is to balance qi in the body. Its most important element, in my opinion, is its self-cultivation and discipline; practitioners learn to control their own qi in order to guide it into patients' bodies. The actual practice of qigong is fairly wide-ranging, however, from those who rely on a tai chi–type movement or yoga to a ritual like that of Master Yang, which has more of a shamanistic bent.

Despite the formidable title of "Master," when I met Yang I was pleasantly surprised to find an elderly Chinese grandmother who hurried us—my husband, Noah, had come along for the ride—into her house and made us dumplings. After we'd chatted and eaten, she started the treatment with a scan. This simply required that we sit in front of her as she "studied us with her consciousness," moving her eyes up and down our bodies. At the end of my scan, she observed there was stagnation in my uterus. I'd recently been diagnosed with polyps in my uterus, so that was impressive. (Though also a fair guess for a perimenopausal woman in her fifties like me.) Then she'd made some ritualistic hand movements and held the palm of her right hand in front of me. On it appeared a small pile of powder. It truly did seem to have just emerged from her palm. I had watched very carefully and yet was still confounded. After giving me the powder and telling me to add water and drink it, she turned to Noah and said he needed something to help him experience more love. (That was a first—it's not a problem I had been aware of for him—but he went with it.) She tapped her thumb and her forefinger together—once, twice, a small dent appeared in her thumb, and, three times, after which a pill appeared between them. This sent me reeling. I had been an inch from Master Yang's hands to watch this as it happened. Still, I couldn't figure out any other way she was doing this than to actually be materializing these things. Her daughter told me that Master Yang never knows what form the herbs will take; sometimes, she produces liquid and everyone has to run off looking for a cup.

I had been so turned around, I'd called Bill Bengston from my hotel room and reported breathlessly: "I've just seen a qigong practitioner in Orange County, California, who made powder and pills magically appear in her hands."

"The correct term," he replied, "is 'materialization.'"

"Wait, you know about this? It's a thing?"

"Oh, sure, there are anthropologists who study it," he said casually. "I thought it was exclusively practiced abroad, though—you say you saw someone in California? Can you bring the powder back with you so we can analyze it in the lab?"

"I drank it," I said—suddenly all too aware of my reckless decision to do so.

I never did get to the bottom of what happened with Master Yang and her spontaneous medicine that day. I couldn't shake the feeling that I'd seen an incredible magic act—which had held me back from committing to the experience fully. But, then, it was almost a relief to feel a bit of doubt. It was the prime mover for my investigation, the very reason for writing this book; I didn't want to lose sight of it.

I did, however, later uncover scientific research into qigong's effectiveness, though nothing that would explain the supernatural conjuring of herbs or medicine. Still, I was curious to find a study[14] on qigong healers conducted in Japan in 1992. Using a magnetometer, researchers had found that the electromagnetic fields surrounding the heads, bodies, and hands of qigong practitioners during breathing meditations were extraordinarily large—about one thousand times larger than the strongest electromagnetic fields, those that surround the heart in humans. This is made more intriguing in the context of work done by the late Dr. Andrew L. Bassett, a professor of orthopedic surgery at the College of Physicians and Surgeons at Columbia University. He and his colleagues, in the face of much skepticism from their peers, showed that pulsing electromagnetic fields could be used to heal fractured limbs. This was based on an earlier discovery that cell functions could be controlled by external electromagnetic fields.[15] (At the time of Bassett's death in 1994, his electromagnetic technique, according to Columbia University, had been used successfully on more than one hundred thousand patients nationwide to heal broken bones that would have otherwise required surgery.)[16] Perhaps, as biologist and biophysicist Dr. James Oschman posits in his book, *Energy Medicine: The Scientific Basis*,[17] the qigong practitioners were able to "emit powerful pulsing biomagnetic fields in the same frequency range that biomedical researchers have identified for jump-starting healing of soft and hard tissue injuries."[18]

Oschman also looks more generally in his book at the research about "hands-off therapies"—which primarily include qigong, Reiki, and therapeutic touch (TT). He cites the work of Dr. John Zimmerman,[19] who measured the magnetic field frequencies of Reiki practitioners and other energy therapists while they worked on clients, and found that they all emitted extremely low frequencies (ELF) from their hands, which is also the optimal electromagnetic frequency that medical researchers identified for stimulating tissue repair. "In essence," concludes Dr. Oschman, "the electromagnetic fields produced by a practitioner's hands can induce current flows in the tissues and cells of individuals who are in close proximity."[20] When I read these research studies, I was reminded of my recent patient, the man who had broken both of his legs in a skiing accident. He had experienced the energy coming out of my hands so strongly it had made his legs shake and, according to his doctors, he made an unusually rapid recovery. Zimmerman's research showed that it was possible that I was inadvertently emitting a similar frequency to the ones being used in orthopedic hospitals to speed up bone healing.

Perhaps this explanation—as with the theory that the connective tissue is affected by acupuncture, causing chemical changes at a cellular level—is the furthest distance science can take us in illuminating the process. Yet there remains also a mysterious element, not unlike the ineffable element in the process that allows Bengston's mice to recover from cancerous injections or Carla's clients to respond to her evoking streams of light or for the lump in a woman's breast treated by Hiroyuki Abe, a monk and energy healer in Japan, to disappear.

I was introduced to the work of Hiroyuki Abe through Dr. Erik Peper, whom I'd met through Dr. Leah Lagos. Peper, a professor at the Institute for Holistic Health Studies at San Francisco State University, had asked Abe, in 2007, to be a guest speaker for his Holistic Health Western Perspectives class. After his lecture, in which Abe described his method, he offered to perform healings on the students. The students' reactions—they were astonished by the improvements they experienced almost immediately—prompted Peper to formally research Abe's healing process. In his follow-up study, Peper found that, after one treatment, 65 percent of thirty students reported a reduction in troublesome symptoms.[21] Three months later, these students reported continued significant benefits as a result of the treatment. And, if students were treated more than once, the results were considerably more pronounced.

Peper, himself, was treated by Abe and found that the limited range of movement in his knee—from a torn medial meniscus he'd suffered nine months prior—was resolved in a single healing session. That session was eleven years ago. Peper and Abe have been in touch since, perhaps most significantly in treating a child of one of Peper's colleagues. In 2013, Peper asked Abe to work with Yuval Oded, an Israeli psychologist, whose son was born with a rare developmental deficiency called corectopia, which means the pupil is displaced in the eye. This condition can cause severe myopia, but, in the case of Yuval's son, it caused blindness in his left eye. By the time the child was ten months old, he had met with and been operated on by a number of prominent doctors, to no avail. Despite their misgivings about energy healing, Yuval and his wife decided to try having Abe treat their son. After a Skype session, in which Abe identified a minor health condition that Yuval's wife suffered though the couple had not mentioned it, they traveled to Japan to meet him in person. "Abe did not touch our child," recalls Yuval of Abe's work with his son, "but mainly moved his hands a few centimeters from him, concentrating very hard and snapping his fingers." The family visited him six more times over the course of their ten-day visit. After the last treatment, they brought their boy outside and he seemed suddenly "dazed and sun-blinded." His sight had been restored. Yuval, whose now four-year-old son has developed wonderfully with vision in both eyes, is still, as he joyously told me, "stunned and very, very grateful" for Abe's treatment. "We now understand," he said, "that healing powers exist beyond our understanding."

When Noah and I arrived at the Osaka airport, Abe was there to receive us with a translator he had brought with him. (He does not speak English and, as I learned, is meticulous about being accurately interpreted. In fact, when he has a particularly nuanced point to convey or is being observed doing his work, Abe brings in a second translator from Tokyo.) Abe is a tall man with a kind face and an avuncular presence. Right away, he requested that we first spend time together, getting to know each other and observing him in clinic, before I interview him about his work. And, with that, he swept us into his orbit, taking us out to a restaurant, giving us a tour of the city, riding with us on the bullet train for a trip to Kyoto. Even with our conversation filtered through a translator, his warmth was palpable. Abe is exuberant, talkative, and funny. He enjoys a freedom with his vices—he drinks and smokes heartily—and was, in short, excellent company. After we'd gotten to know each other socially, he allowed me to observe his work for two days at a clinic run by one of his students in a suburb outside of Kobe. (Abe visits there occasionally to work with patients whom the student, working as a healer, or his staff of acupuncturists are having trouble helping.) It was a wonderful whirlwind—and, true to his word, we did not discuss the nature of his work until it was over.

By the time we finally did sit down to discuss his healing practice, I'd gleaned at least a bit about his background from our earlier outings. Abe grew up in a city just west of Tokyo in a close-knit family with his father and mother and older sister. He lost his father when he was six years old. Just after his father died, his mother was diagnosed with brain cancer. A female monk in the neighborhood who had been trained to heal people began to visit his mother. She wrote sutras on paper, according to Abe, and asked his mother to swallow the paper. As a small boy, he remembers watching his mom eat the paper like medicine, literally swallowing the lessons of Buddhism imparted to her by the monk. And, amazingly, his mother got better over the course of four years. She had no conventional medical treatment; she was prescribed only herbal medicine, drunk as a tea, and small wads of paper. This made a strong impression on Abe. He developed a sense of spirituality and a strong belief in the power of prayer since, as a young boy, he had prayed for his mother to live.

He did not go to college but attended a technical school for two years and then worked in construction in his twenties. His religious faith never wavered, but he didn't yet feel a sense of purpose in his life. He married young and, by the time he was nearing thirty, the marriage began to fall apart. On his thirtieth birthday, he went to visit his mother and told her the sad news that his relationship was coming to an end. While sitting with her drinking tea, he suddenly saw an apparition of a goddess. She had a beautiful face and was wearing a typical monk's robe. He looked to his mother for a reaction, but it was clear that she could not see the goddess. In the end, he decided not to mention this to his mother, he told me with a laugh, because he "didn't want to have to give her any more strange news after telling her about my divorce."

The goddess, Abe learned, was the Shinto goddess of mercy. She has been by his side ever since. Shintoism, alongside Buddhism, is the traditional religion of Japan, though "Shinto" also has different meanings for people in Japan; some simply visit Shinto shrines without being devoutly religious. But most everyone believes in *kami*, which encompasses the sacred spirits that take the form of things—the wind, mountains, trees, and rivers—and concepts, like fertility or a sense of wonder. Kami, however, also refers to the many gods—more than eight hundred thousand—that Shintos worship. In this context, it is less unusual for a goddess to have appeared to Abe and to have remained as a presence in his life, talking with him as she does, and guiding him.

Peper offers additional insight about the influence of religion and belief systems on the ways in which healers shape their practices. "Healers channel . . . and then they adapt it—'it' meaning the power to heal—to their own cultural beliefs," he says. "So if you're Christian, it might be Mary. Abe sees a goddess. The process is the same, but the expression that comes out is encoded in your cultural bias."[22] Peper suggests that this cultural bias also extends to the ceremony of healing. "If you talk to Native American healers, they spend days fasting and bowing and . . . smoking, you name it, but those are simply rituals to evoke that place where you feel centered and open."[23]

It was the goddess who led Abe to healing. The first time that he healed someone—a woman who was a swimmer with arthritis in her back and joints—he was instructed by the goddess to do so. She told him what to do—including the distinct movements he makes with his hands to this day, snapping and tapping in combination—and the woman did indeed feel her pain dissipate. "Are you sure?" Abe asked her repeatedly throughout the treatment. As he spoke of this, I thought back to my early days in clinic and the disbelief I felt when my patients made measurable progress. This feeling had prompted the journey that found me here, sitting in Kobe, talking to this man, now a healer with enough experience to have a quiet confidence in his abilities.

Over time, he learned how to develop and hone his ability. He started to experience visions as he treated his patients, as if he could see into their bodies. Muscle glowed red; bone appeared as gleaming white. But he wanted to be able to offer more substantial explanations to his patients, who had started to come to him through word of mouth. So he began to study anatomy, physiology, pathology. He immersed himself in medical textbooks. All the while, the goddess helped him, too, offering insights and direction as he practiced, sometimes arguing with him. ("She was bossy and old-school," Abe amusingly complained to me of the time after she had first arrived, when they were often in conflict.)

As he gained insight into the functions of the body and how it heals, he began to take on students. It is common in Asia for master healers to have apprentices, as the tradition is that skills are passed on by initiation. (A similar model is used to teach Reiki, which is also a Japanese practice.) He says he is able to offer a kind of accelerated start to his students—by performing a powerful chakra-opening ceremony that removes some of the impediments to channeling—and then it is up to them to develop from there. His view of healing is surprisingly didactic in that he believes everyone can learn and that practice, not intuition or enlightenment, is what makes someone a better healer. He also believes that all of his students have guides, as he does, but that not all of them are able to connect as strongly with them. I met three of his students while I was there; all of them spoke admiringly, and gratefully, of the lessons Abe has taught them.

One of these students runs the clinic just outside Kobe that I visited to observe Abe work. Here, I watched as he saw a little more than a dozen patients in a day, several of whom he'd treated before. All of them came in with complaints of pain— fibromyalgia, lower back aches, frozen shoulder—and, after Abe went to work with his clicking and tapping, identifying the pain and directing his energy, they all said they were relieved of their suffering to a substantial degree. What fascinated me was that I noticed that Abe usually worked along the same points and meridians I do—only he was tapping instead of administering needles.

When a woman in her fifties came in complaining of a frozen shoulder, Abe identified scoliosis in her spine. He put his palm on her shoulder and, with his other hand, tapped the acupuncture points around her left scapula. When he sensed his power diminishing in this treatment, he prayed to his guide. Finally, he asked me to give the patient acupuncture as I would normally to treat a frozen shoulder. When I put the needles in at the lower part of her leg, Abe put his hand over mine and ran energy down my finger into the needle. I felt an instant and intense ache in my hand, and a vibrating sensation like I've never felt.

While this physical experience certainly validated to me that Abe had electric hands, what solidified his authenticity in my mind was that most of his patients healed gradually over time, and he tended to treat rather mundane problems. Lightning did not strike in every session. It was a therapeutic relationship—often with two steps forward, one step back—and therefore more subtle, and real, than a miraculous stunt. Abe, too, possesses an earthbound modesty about his work. "You'll meet many healers who say they have a guide," he told me. "Please use me as a baseline when evaluating their skills. I am of a lower rank, so if they can't work at my level, they are probably frauds."

And yet Peper described Abe as a healer at the next level, working in a state that many others are still striving to reach. "When he is there, he is there. He may drink and smoke—I like to call him my nicotine healer—but when he is with the person he is healing, he is totally centered and at rest. You feel totally accepted. There is no threat. And, by mirror imaging, in a sense, you evoke that centered state too. You're reducing your anxiety, your panic, all your thoughts. At that moment, that is when healing occurs."[24]

On our last night together, Abe took us out to dinner at a shabu-shabu restaurant—where the elements of this Japanese hot pot dish are cooked in cast-iron pots at the table—with a group of his students. We all sat cross-legged on tatami mats, pressed together at a tiny table, everyone throwing different ingredients into the pot at the center of the table. Midway through the dinner, as everyone was drinking and laughing, I began to suffer one of my bouts of tachycardia. (With my heart condition, this is always a possibility, but I believe in this case, it was precipitated by an attunement Abe had given me earlier that day, which I'll describe in Chapter 10.) At that point, these episodes had occurred rarely enough that I was no longer carrying beta-blockers with me. I began to discreetly do vagal maneuvers—bearing down while attempting to massage the carotid artery in my neck—to try to reduce the speed of my heart. It was a futile effort, and I began to panic. I had visions of being raced to the hospital in Japan, where I'd have to have my heart stopped and restarted again with adenosine. As my heart began to beat more rapidly and my brain was increasingly deprived of oxygen, I started to feel faint. Pressed in among Abe's students, getting jostled as they threw vegetables into the pot and stirred the ingredients, I was miserable. I looked at Noah and quietly indicated that I was struggling. Abe caught sight of our exchange. He leaned toward Noah, conferring with him in murmurs across the table. Then he looked at me, pointed two fingers at me, and shook them once, as if he were shooting an imaginary gun at my heart. Immediately, my heart went back into a normal rhythm.

The next day, still reeling a bit from the spectacular experience of the night before, I said goodbye to Abe, who came to send Noah and me off at the train station in Kobe, and we began our travels to Fukuoka, on the northern shore of the Japanese island of Kyushu. I felt enriched by my time with Abe—he was someone I had truly learned from in a spiritual and humane way. As I turned from him—literally; he stood on the train platform, waving until the bitter end—I looked ahead toward my next meeting. I was, again on Peper's recommendation and generous introduction, going to meet Master Mitsumasa Kawakami, another healer of great acclaim, in part because of his severe displays of self-mastery, which included piercing his tongue with a skewer. Peper had sent me photos and a short video of this beforehand, and the violent image had been hovering in my mind ever since. To be honest, I was still uncertain as to how this connected to healing—it seemed, in fact, to fiercely contradict it—but, as the train whisked us forward, I knew I was inexorably headed toward finding out.

YOU THE HEALER

A Chakra Meditation

- The supernatural experiences that both Carla and Abe describe are the result of a spiritual preparation that requires much discipline and clarity. Their experiences are also informed by their beliefs. Like Erik Peper, I believe that healers all channel the same source energy, but how they perceive it depends on their belief system. Despite these differences, most healers (including both Carla and Abe) experience the chakras as powerful energy centers, and this meditation is designed to acquaint you with yours.

- Each chakra is associated with a specific color. Color is simply a wave traveling through space. Depending on the wavelength, our eyes register different colors. Visualizing a particular color can prompt your body to simulate that color's wavelength.

- Sit quietly with a straight spine and focus on breathing deep into your abdomen.

- Send your grounding laser from the area around the base of your spine deep into the earth.

- Visualize the crown chakra at the top of your head. Imagine violet light passing through the top of your head and permeating your body. The crown chakra is associated with faith, trust, inspiration, and our connection to source. When this chakra is open, your head will feel open and airy, and you will experience a feeling of joy and expansiveness.

- As you feel this chakra open up, turn your attention to the middle of your forehead, imagining the area as a dark indigo-blue light. This is the third-eye chakra, and when it is open it gives us clarity, wisdom, spiritual insight, and sometimes clairvoyance.

- Once you have felt this chakra fully, move your attention

to your throat and imagine light blue light passing through the area. The throat chakra is about confidence, truth, and expression.

- Move from the throat to the area around the heart, imagining a funnel of green light moving in and out of your chest. The heart chakra is the center of love, connection with others, forgiveness, compassion, and generosity.

- Next comes the solar plexus chakra, which is located in the upper abdomen (in about the same place as you feel butterflies in the stomach, which is appropriate because this is the chakra related to our gut feelings and emotions). In your mind, run yellow light through this chakra, clearing out residual pain.

- The sacral chakra is in your lower abdomen, and it responds to orange light, so go ahead and visualize the chakra as orange. It's associated with our sexuality and creativity, as well as our identity in the world.

- The final chakra is the root chakra, which is located at the bottom of the spine. You can strengthen it by sending red light to the area. As the chakra closest to the earth, it is associated with grounding, resilience, and physical survival.

7

MYSTICS AMONG US

When we arrived at the Kawakami Slow Yoga Studio in Fukuoka, a party was in full swing. Master Kawakami had mentioned to me that there would be a small gathering at his studio in celebration of the upcoming publication of his sixteenth book, a psychological exploration of the young Buddha—he'd failed to mention, however, that it would be a lavish affair, with singing and dancing performed by Kawakami himself, followed by a five-course meal at a nearby Italian restaurant. I was woefully underdressed and a bit worn from traveling, but I was also getting good at going with the flow of this adventure. So I found my place at the dinner table—I had been graciously seated next to the guest of honor—and settled in.

In contrast to the rather startling images that had been running through my mind of Kawakami with a skewer plunged through his tongue, I was delighted to encounter one of the most joyous and unselfconscious humans I have ever met. He took my hand as he sat down next to me at dinner, dressed nattily in a navy-blue pin-striped suit with a purple tie and matching pocket square, and looked at me warmly. "I know of the pain that your mother caused you as a child," he told me through his translator, and then added that he was sorry that she had passed away. As these were not details of my life he could have discovered through an Internet search, I found his words both comforting and unsettling. I smiled and nodded in response, quietly hoping that I'd learn over time how he'd acquired this information.

Kawakami then introduced me to his team at the yoga center, each one bearing small gifts for me (and Noah as well), including a purse that one woman had woven from the fabric of her mother's kimono. (The Japanese culture, I learned time and again on this trip, is benevolent first and foremost; we were frequently bowing in gratitude for gifts, helpful advice, shared meals, wisdom imparted to us.) Several of the people I met introduced themselves as Kawakami's apprentices. When I asked Kawakami what they were learning, he explained that they were practicing "channeling" on behalf of the patients. This, as I would later observe in person, meant that they were helping patients by receiving information through automatic writing. This information was deemed as critical in helping healer and patient understand the soul's purpose and the past lives, which informed their present-day struggles. The idea of past lives is a central tenet in Buddhism as well as in Kawakami's practice: he believes that our current lives are inextricably linked with former ones. "Unless a person clears the trauma from their past, they cannot become enlightened," he told me, explaining that in order to be truly expansive, to understand how broadly we exist in the world—which is to say beyond personal consciousness—we need to let go of painful experiences from our current and previous lives that inhibit us. This is essentially another view on Chinese medicine's stagnation or Kiran's "dense energetic forms" or the cellular memory, as discussed in Chapter 3, that biologists at UCLA have been researching. For Kawakami, this state is necessary for both the patient and the healer; the patient must contend with old suffering to achieve better health, and the healer must do so in order to achieve the stillness, and selflessness, necessary to help.

Channeling information from source energy—or what Kawakami would call a "soul reading"—is the first, and lengthy, step in the process of becoming a healer in Kawakami's practice (many of his apprentices are still practicing this critical step after twenty years of training; it is difficult to move beyond because healing requires attaining a level of selflessness, or unattached ego, that Kawakami believes requires decades of practice). In addition to the reckoning with past lives, working toward optimum physical and mental health are also essential components of Kawakami's holistic program. Kawakami, himself, at seventy-nine years old, is committed to a rigorous diet and exercise regimen; he does not smoke, he takes one alcoholic drink a week, and he lifts weights, practices yoga, and meditates every day. (This made for an intriguing contrast with Hiroyuki Abe, who drank and smoked freely throughout the time I'd spent with him the week before.) Toward the end of the night, a stylish young woman, her hair in a tight, shoulder-length bob, introduced herself to me. She told me she was a psychologist working alongside Kawakami and his apprentices. Her job, Kawakami explained, was to help his patients change unhealthy mental patterns so they could become more open and responsive to his healing. By the end of my first night, I'd already garnered some insight into the unique approach—both mystical and methodical at once—that Kawakami brings to his healing practice.

Kawakami was born in 1938 in Nagasaki, which, after centuries of Japan's isolation due to strict regulations on commerce and foreign relations, was one of the few cities that had communication with the rest of the world. The nearby island of Dejima—literally meaning "Exit Island"—had been the only post for direct trade and exchange with other countries. As a boy, living near Dejima, Kawakami met a diverse group of people who came from an array of backgrounds and religious traditions. His father, who was a captain of a merchant ship, traveled frequently. Kawakami says his father, too, offered different ideas and ways of seeing the world. As we talked, Kawakami pulled from his wallet a picture of his father, who is no longer alive: it was an image of a handsome man in a captain's hat with an etched and thoughtful face. "He was never angry or scolded me," Kawakami said appreciatively.

His mother—whom he does not, as he pointed out, carry a picture of in his wallet—was very strict. She was also, however, a devout Buddhist and taught Kawakami important spiritual lessons. As part of her religious instruction, she taught Kawakami that he should help other people and make a contribution to society. When, as a child, he wondered what his reward for such contributions might be, she emphasized the importance of giving freely and without expectation. (This lesson was brought into stark relief in 1945, when Kawakami was six years old, and the United States dropped an atomic bomb on Nagasaki. Gratefully, by then, Kawakami and his family were living in Hirado, about forty-six miles from Nagasaki, but he remembers seeing "the flash of the bomb and the mushroom cloud" from a distance. Afterward, his mother's lesson—give to others without restraint—was impressed upon him more strenuously.) Sometimes, as a small boy, his mother would bathe him outside, in a deep barrel tub, as is customary to do in Japan. She would put a leaf in the water just out of her son's reach. When he struggled to grasp it, it would often sink or float away, but when he sat calmly, she taught him to gently move the current of the water so that the leaf would flow toward him naturally. "Where there is a will, there is a way," she would say, explaining that this is often accomplished by finding stillness as opposed to creating struggle.

But she also delivered an unintended spiritual message to her son when one day Kawakami, while playing, broke his mother's beloved statue of Buddha. She was furious and warned him that there would be dire consequences for harming Buddha in this way. He waited and waited. At first, he was terrified, but, when he realized that nothing was actually going to happen, that there would be no otherworldly punishment, he was set free. His mother had been wrong. At that moment, he stopped believing in the superstitions that often accompany religious beliefs.

Kawakami is something of a celebrity in Japan. Today, he is known for his healing ability, but he first rose to prominence in 1972, when he was named Mr. Japan in their first-ever official bodybuilding competition. (He later went on to be a contestant in the Mr. Universe competition.) There were no gyms in Japan at the time. Fascinated by the bodybuilders in America, Kawakami trained himself with weights and equipment he made himself, modeling them on the ones he'd seen in *Strength and Health*[1] magazine (which he translated on his own in order to read the articles). There are, as he showed me, photos from this time of a young, astonishingly muscular Kawakami with an arm thrown round Arnold Schwarzenegger.

Kawakami enjoyed the hard work of bodybuilding and realized his own energetic drive in doing it, but, at a certain point, he felt that he was hitting a wall. He wanted to expand his training, to push himself toward higher concentration and focus. When Kawakami was thirty-three years old, he participated in an international bodybuilding contest in Iraq, where he met an Indian bodybuilder named Monotosh Roy. The two became fast friends. Over time, Roy became Kawakami's master, teaching him to go beyond the aggressiveness of bodybuilding into the highly disciplined, more meditative practice of yoga. Soon, Kawakami abandoned bodybuilding altogether and devoted himself to the study of yoga. He was captivated by the single-mindedness of the effort, the complete absorption required of his mind and body. Where he had once been all forceful determination, he felt now that he was gaining steadier control over his body while, at the same time, deepening his meditative abilities. These two attributes—command of his body and mental quietude—would become central to Kawakami's philosophy and practice.

From his yoga practice, he developed a breathing method of

his own, in which he takes two breaths per minute for a period of twenty minutes, reducing his heart rate as well as inhibiting his reactions to internal and external stimuli. (Once, he undertook this exercise at a doctor's office; when the nurse tried to take his pulse, she couldn't find it.) Kawakami became so secure while doing this type of breathing, and felt so profoundly pacified during it, he came to see it as a state of enlightenment. "I am able to attain a spiritual state of perfect stillness," he told me, "and while doing so, I can control my five senses so I don't feel anything."[2] Taking his own unique route, Kawakami achieves a transcendence that others such as Kiran, Bill, and Abe have also described: he no longer feels the separation of self because he has fully united with source.

It is at this point in the story that the skewers through the tongue come into play. In order to test his ability to expand his consciousness, Kawakami began to submit himself to brutal acts of self-mutilation. Once he'd reached a profound meditative state, for example, he'd hold his tongue with one hand while pushing a skewer through it with the other—and he discovered that he did not feel any pain while doing so.

"The only way you really know if you have control of your consciousness is in some sense to test yourself," muses Peper, who has observed Kawakami in his lab several times as he has done this. "When he found that he could pierce himself, he knew that he had really mastered the skill. It's not so different from when he became Mr. Japan. In essence, he is like any true athlete, or meditator, in that he developed this practice over time and, as a result, he now has an extraordinary level of control."[3]

In addition to Peper's study of Kawakami[4]—during which

he was hooked up to an EKG and EEG, both of which showed that Kawakami had almost no physical reactivity as the skewer went through his tongue—he was also studied by researchers in Japan, who burned his feet with medical lasers (ordinarily used to burn tissue) as he lay motionless in an MRI. They, too, found that pain did not register in his brain. Drawing a blood sample from Kawakami afterward, however, they discovered a significant increase in his endorphins, suggesting that his body had responded to pain by producing its own natural painkillers, even as his brain had failed to register the *sensation* of pain.

Though even Kawakami cannot offer an explanation for this altered state—the act was born out of, and is practiced as, pure instinct—Peper believes there are two components that help to decipher the phenomenon. "He has no anticipation of fear [as the skewer goes in] . . . Somewhere deep in his mind, he feels totally safe," Peper hypothesizes. "And the second part: he uses breathing as the mechanism to not have pain, to control, and to not react."[5]

The idea that Kawakami's breath might help him block pain returns us, in fact, to Dr. Lagos's discussion of heart rate variability, the measure of the variation in time between heartbeats. Lagos, as described in Chapter 2, teaches her patients breathing exercises with the goal of helping them develop the "ability to control their physiology and psychology through their heart rhythms."[6] By altering the body's autonomic nervous system—which encompasses the body's sympathetic (fight-or-flight) and parasympathetic (calming) reactions—through breath, Lagos's patients are able to modify their response to stress. Kawakami, though admittedly an extreme case, is essentially employing the

same mechanism. On his inhale, when he is sympathetically activated, he stops any movement; in the middle of his exhale, when
there is an increase of parasympathetic activity or, as Peper describes it, "regeneration," he pierces his body with the skewer. In
the exhalation phase, in other words, he doesn't feel injury. (Here,
I feel compelled to say: please don't try this at home! Kawakami,
needless to say, is a rare creature, the likes of which I have never
before seen and perhaps never will see again.) Clearly, there is a
complex interweaving of physiological and psychological—and
even spiritual—prompts that allows Kawakami to painlessly endure such a feat. But I believe that his breathing technique, and
the control he has gained over his nervous system, play a critical
role not only in developing this endurance but also in his capacity as a healer.

Kawakami's control over his body and mind allows him the space
he needs to heal others. By expanding his own consciousness, he
explained, he is able to access a clear vision of a patient's needs
as well as a direct path to the energy required to heal. While his
technique appears drastic, in reality it is simply a variation on
what every healer in this book, myself included, describes as a
necessary condition required to help others: that is, to surrender
the perception of a separate self.

Kawakami also stresses the importance of maintaining a steady
emotional equilibrium. The daily intrusions of the mind that most
of us feel—be it from anxiety or rage or sadness—keep us, and
our energy, rooted in a narrow, isolated consciousness. It is this
separateness that leads to the kinds of problems that Kawakami

calls a "spiritual emergency," an emotional or physical breakdown that forces a person to confront both past and present suffering.

It is at this juncture that people tend to seek out Kawakami for guidance and healing. In his sessions, as described earlier, his apprentices aid patients in accessing information from their past lives through automatic writing; sometimes the patients, too, are asked to write. While in Fukuoka, I observed Kawakami work with a young woman with an eczema-like skin condition covering much of her body. She lay down on a mat on the floor and closed her eyes. Kawakami laid his hands on the parts of her body where her condition was most concentrated and began to sing. The sound he emitted was, at first, piercing—like a low-level alarm—but it was also a pure tone, classically shamanistic in its quality. "It's hard to have any thoughts present at the same time when you hear it next to you," Peper once remarked to me of Kawakami's singing. "It almost erases thoughts and worries because you're overwhelmed by the tone." I thought it was an astute point. That is, as we become increasingly absorbed in a sound, particularly one that requires concentration in order to adjust to it, we are also diverting our attention from mistrust or defensiveness or self-consciousness, all feelings that otherwise might keep us from opening to a healing session. (I will explore the use of sound in healing in more detail in Chapter 9.) The young woman shut her eyes and remained very still. Kawakami handed the woman a clipboard and pen. Without opening her eyes, as if she were in a trance, she began to write a story. It was an account, Kawakami's translator told me, of her previous life when she had been a man who worked as a doctor. She had been very successful and a rival physician had poured boiling oil on her hand in a jealous fit. The skin of her hand had become putrid and infested with insects.

"Physiologically, if you observe the brain of Kawakami or his apprentices, or even the patients when they are being treated by Kawakami, when they are doing automatic writing, you see that they are in a more receptive mode during this time," says Peper, who did in fact hook up some of Kawakami's apprentices to an EEG as they were automatic writing. "At that moment, they are not orienting outward or reacting to stimuli. They get so quiet, they get rid of themselves, they are passively open; that is part of the yogic practice. Whatever messages come in, that is what they write down. I think people can learn to do this."[7] Indeed they can: this is essentially what Neale Donald Walsch did when he wrote *Conversations with God*.

Kawakami discovered his own past lives, as he tells it, when he meditated for twenty-nine days straight and then instinctively began to write. He felt that he was directly accessing information at large in the universe. He learned that his spirit's destiny has always been to help people; this, he believes, has played out over many lifetimes and incarnations. "I've had the same job for five thousand years," he told me. The experience crystallized for him the notion that other incarnations stay with us and that his role is to heal accumulated trauma and pain as a route to happiness.

"I would say as you develop in meditational practice, you develop psychic skills. As Kawakami [developed his meditation] . . . and developed a deep empathy, he became aware of consciousness [at] its multiple levels, which I don't totally understand, if I'm being honest," Peper says of Kawakami's automatic writing experience. "I am sure it is true for him—what I mean is his

interpretation of that energetic reality—that is the model he created because it fits his cultural conditioning. I've certainly seen
him do some remarkable things." To me, automatic writing is
another expression of having removed the filter between a person and the larger energy field. There are certainly a lot of traps
with this practice—I've seen people believe they are automatic
writing when in fact it was their subconscious or ego bubbling
up—but I believe that it is also possible to hit a groove, such as
Neale did, such as Kawakami does, and begin to transcribe information that is afloat in the field. Authentic automatic writing
is not unlike creative inspiration, when a person has unfettered
access to ideas or wisdom or even instruction in the larger energy
field. Incidentally, I now believe that Kawakami was performing a kind of mental version of automatic writing when we first
met and he spoke of the sadness my mother had caused me as a
child; he is certainly one of the most evolved healers I have ever
met—he generates an overwhelming sense of warmth and safety
as a result—and it does not surprise me that he'd be able to retrieve information about others in this way.

What struck me most about Kawakami was that his fierce discipline is not about asceticism or deprivation. It is, in fact, about
expansion. Though mind-expanding and consciousness-hacking
exercises have recently become fashionable ("Everyone is trying to
alter their consciousness,"[8] as one young business entrepreneur put
it recently)—giving rise to mindfulness apps and sensory deprivation tanks—these are generally motivated by a desire to increase
performance and happiness (as well as build businesses) whereas,

in the case of Kawakami, it is an endeavor to relinquish his sense of self, rather than enhance it. His yoga and breathing and meditation practices are a means to an end: to connect to the larger energy field. The evidence of this is boldly on display in his ability to endure self-inflicted injury but also, more subtly, in his peaceful temperament and his strength as a healer. Most healing traditions involve increasing awareness, or accessing another realm, but often this is at least partly done with the aid of hallucinogens. Shamans, for example, take ayahuasca, a brew made from natural ingredients, including the ayahuasca vine (*Banisteriopsis caapi*) and a shrub called chacruna (*Psychotria viridis*).[9] The brew contains the hallucinogenic drug dimethyltryptamine (DMT), sometimes referred to as the spirit molecule, because it induces spiritual experiences.[*] To induce their mystical state, Native Americans take peyote, made from a small, spineless cactus with psychoactive alkaloids, namely mescaline (which causes hallucinogenic effects similar to LSD and psilocybin mushrooms). Western medicine, too, is beginning to recognize the therapeutic value of hallucinogens: over the last decade, "microdosing" small quantities of these drugs has come to be considered a beneficial practice in many circles. Researchers have begun to test the effects of the drug psilocybin[10] (by taking patients through well-guided "trips" in clin-

---

[*] Our bodies are capable of producing DMT naturally. One of the most fascinating, and controversial, explanations of near-death experiences was posited by Dr. Rick Strassman, clinical associate professor of psychiatry at the University of New Mexico School of Medicine, who, in the 1990s, proposed that DMT is released in large quantities from the pineal gland in the hours before we die and when we are born. Depending on your point of view, this means that either DMT connects us to spirit at the times when we are entering and leaving the world (which is how a shaman would see it) or that DMT induces a spiritual "trip" that gives the illusion of being connected to something greater.

ical settings with soothing music and therapists on hand) in the
hope that it could be used to effectively treat an array of mental
health disorders, such as depression, addiction, and anxiety. In
a clinical trial at UCLA,[11] twelve late-stage cancer patients were
found to have a significant reduction in anxiety for three months
after taking the drug, and the improvement in mood lasted for up
to six months. In trials for a study at Johns Hopkins University,
which were published in 2006,[12] 2008,[13] and 2011,[14] varying doses
of psilocybin were given to thirty-six "healthy, normal" subjects
with a spiritual orientation of some kind (ranging from attend-
ing church or synagogue to participating in a meditation group).
At the fourteen-month follow-up in the 2011 study, 94 percent
of volunteers ranked their high-dose experience among the five
most spiritually significant experiences of their lives; 83 percent
reported that it had increased their overall sense of well-being.
Robin Carhart-Harris, a psychopharmacologist and the lead author of studies on the psychedelic from the Imperial College of
London, used an MRI to track movement in the brain when under the influence of psilocybin.[15] Carhart-Harris's team discovered
that the drug decreases activity in two areas: the medial prefrontal
cortex (mPFC) and the posterior cingulated cortex (PCC). The
mPFC is known to be more active during depression, and the
PCC is understood to play a role in consciousness and self-identity.
Carhart-Harris explains: "Heightened activity in this [network of
the brain] correlates with excessive introspection, being stuck in
one's own head and detached from the outside world."[16]

While his methods are different—and do not require hallu-

cinogens of any kind—this is exactly what Kawakami is able
to achieve: letting go of identity with all of its pain and dis-
tractions. And with this also comes a dramatic ability to allow
energy, or information, from the larger field to come through.
I came away from my time with Kawakami feeling that he was
living proof that we have more potential for healing ourselves
and others than we might ever imagine—not to mention that it
is possible to open our minds to information in the energy field
without hallucinogens, natural or otherwise. It is remarkably
challenging to submit to new experiences, particularly when
they are uncomfortable and require adjusting our attitude about
well-worn conventions—but the outcome can be incredible.
Peper describes Kawakami's attitude in this way: "His innate
response is 'Let's explore and see.'"[17] I saw that in Kawakami
too; there is a crucial uninhibitedness within his discipline. This
supreme openness, coupled with an unyielding commitment to
his regimen and a desire to help others, has offered him seemingly limitless possibility.

YOU THE HEALER

Circular Breathing

Master Kawakami's healing skills rely on his ability to control
his breath. He expands his consciousness by breathing unusually
slowly. For those of us without his skills, speeding up our breath
slightly can give us a glimpse of how breathing techniques can

alter consciousness and make us more receptive to information from the broader field.

- Lie down on your back, relax, and practice the resonant breathing exercise from Chapter 2, breathing in for a count of six and out for a count of six.
- Once you feel calm and relaxed, begin to change your breathing patterns. Slowly breathe in through your nose, allowing the air to expand your lungs and move your abdomen outward. At the end of your inhale, immediately begin to exhale through your mouth, keeping the speed the same. At the end of your exhale, immediately begin breathing in through your nose again, slowly and steadily.
- Focus on this circular breathing, making sure you are not holding your breath. There should be no gap between the inhale and the exhale, so when your lungs are almost full, begin to exhale, and when they are almost empty, begin to inhale again.
- As you repeat this circular breathing, you will notice that you're breathing a little faster than usual, but be careful not to speed up too much. I'm not trying to get you to hyperventilate, and you should not feel anxious. On the contrary, this exercise should feel effortless, and your body should feel calm and relaxed.
- At around the ten-minute mark, you may begin to feel your consciousness shift. Some people describe the feeling as euphoric or tingly. At this point you may feel unusually receptive to inspiration.

- Stop after twenty minutes and spend a few minutes breathing normally. It is usually at this point that I feel the most connected to source. Write down any thoughts that come to you. They are often very revealing.

This exercise can make some people feel light-headed. Don't attempt it if you are unwell and especially if you are pregnant or suffer from high blood pressure or cardiovascular disease.

8

WHAT'S IN A PLACEBO?

A few years ago, I visited a renowned healer in New York City. I'd heard about his feats for more than a decade, though the buzz had faded over time. He arrived at the height of his powers in the eighties and was best known for a particular energy that ushered forth from his hands as he passed them over his patients' bodies. The sensation, as people described it to me, seemed like nothing I'd ever experienced. They painted a picture that seemed nothing short of sorcery, and used words like "crackle" and "fierce" and "sharp." When I finally went to see this healer—an elderly man, at that point, in a crowded office with floor-to-ceiling pictures of him standing next to celebrities from his heyday (Melanie Griffith, Don Johnson, and Barbra Streisand among them)—I confess I, too, was dazzled. As he hovered his hands about six inches above my body, I felt a palpable—and, yes, crackling—electricity. As this strange current coursed through me, the healer told me about his life.

Nearly forty years before, he said, slipping into the easy tone of a well-trod story, aliens had abducted him. He did not remember what happened while he was with them, but, when he was released, he discovered that he had the ability to conjure the energy that was now coming out of his hands. He soon learned that his electric touch was also a healing touch, and, once those that he'd helped began to spread his story, people from all walks of life began to flock to him. Bewildered by his account—and the fact that, as he spoke, I felt as if I were a record that he was scratching a needle across—I left the healer's office in a stupor.

As I traveled down the west side of Manhattan, from his office to mine, I thought about his improbable story coupled with his assured ability to channel such vigorous energy. I could see how people might be swept away by the whole experience: the dramatic backstory and the strange but undeniable sensation emitted from his hands. But what, I thought, if that is all there is? What if this man can indeed generate some kind of surging energy that others can feel, and then he tells them about his sensational encounter and the abandon—and promise—of it all convinces his patients that they are being healed? And, in response, they actually *do* heal?

Then, I realized, I might as well be asking the same question of myself. What if I, too, was simply convincing my patients of my abilities? The thought made me extremely uncomfortable. For starters, I wasn't quite ready to throw in my lot with someone who'd told me he'd been captured by aliens. But more seriously, I recoiled at the thought that my work might amount to little more than a psychological trick, or a placebo. As with anyone else in the health-care profession, I'd been rigorously trained to view the placebo effect—meaning a beneficial result produced by an inactive drug or a treatment that occurs due to a patient's belief in its power—as something to avoid. In a research setting, scientists strive to control for the placebo effect, isolating it when possible in order to know the "real" consequence of a treatment versus the consequence of suggestion.

This idea—that I, myself, might be merely a placebo—gave me such a start that I dove into the research on the placebo effect and didn't come back up until I was prepared to give a TED talk on the subject. Which, incidentally, I did do, at the TEDGlobal conference in Edinburgh in 2012.

Before I could proceed with any judgments about placebos, I had to better understand the role they play in healing. As I soon discovered, the placebo has had a bad rap ever since the concept came into being. The word "placebo" is derived from the Latin for "I will please." When, in medieval times, mourners were hired to participate in vespers for the dead, they often chanted a line from Psalm 116: "I shall please the dead in the land of the living."[1] However, as these mourners were merely acting the part, they were considered insincere and people called them "placebos." The term carried over into the medical realm: in the late eighteenth century, it was used to describe a commonplace method or medicine. Over time the definition shifted, and by 1811 "placebo" was defined as "any medicine adapted more to please than to benefit the patient."[2]

In the world of medicine today, a placebo is generally defined as a treatment—such as a pill or an injection or a procedure—

that has a harmless effect and, usually, is proffered unbeknownst to the patient. Interestingly, research has shown that even the appearance of a placebo can influence a patient's reported reaction to it. For example, the larger the pill, the stronger the placebo effect, and two pills elicit a stronger effect than one. Patients have a more positive reaction to brand-name pills than generic ones, and the most powerful responses result from placebos administered by needle.[3] Even the color of placebo pills can alter the outcome: blue ones are more effective than red ones for helping people sleep, and green pills are preferred for anxiety.[4] These are just the kinds of capricious details that have historically made scientists and doctors scoff at the placebo, dismissing it as a trivial mind game.

And yet, despite its negative association, the placebo has played a deceptively positive role in our lives. It has been understood from the start to have a psychologically gratifying, albeit superficial, effect. In 1955, however, Henry Beecher, an anesthesiologist, medical ethicist, and professor at Harvard Medical School, published an influential paper titled "The Powerful Placebo,"[5] which shifted our awareness, if not our bias, about the placebo. Beecher put forth the simple but radical notion that our emotions and beliefs can significantly alter our perception of pain and that the benefit and effectiveness of placebos—used more often at that time, he pointed out, than any other class of drugs—must be recognized.

Beecher's prescient consideration of placebos was bolstered by a study designed more than two decades later by three scientists at the University of California at San Francisco: Jon Levine, Newton Gordon, and Howard Fields. They proposed investigat-

ing whether endorphins—a group of hormones secreted in the
brain and nervous system that activate the body's opiate receiver,
meaning they act as natural painkillers—offered a biochemical
explanation for the placebo effect. As such, the three scientists
told people recovering from dental surgery that they were about
to receive a dose of morphine, saline, or a drug that might increase their pain. The last two drugs, unbeknownst to the patients, were both placebos.

Ultimately, the researchers dismissed those who'd received
morphine and divided the remaining participants into those
who'd responded to the placebos and those who had not. All
of these participants were given Naloxone, a synthetic drug that
blocks opiate receptors in the nervous system, through IV drips.
Naloxone is used to halt overdoses of heroin and morphine—
but it will also block the pain-relieving effect of endorphins.
And, indeed, those participants who'd responded positively to
the placebo suddenly felt an increase in pain when they received
the Naloxone. When the Naloxone was administered to those
who'd not responded to the placebo, they felt no change in their
pain. This was revolutionary: it was the first study to suggest
that placebos can incite chemical responses in the brain similar
to those of active drugs. With that, placebos were no longer only
psychologically significant but also, as with all medication, physiologically too. (It is worth noting that Kawakami, in a sense, became his own placebo: he, too, flooded his body with endorphins
when he was painlessly skewering his tongue.) Subsequent studies using brain scan technology have since confirmed the UCSF
finding and subsequent researchers, most notably neuroscientist
Fabrizio Benedetti at the University of Turin, have shown that

placebos have a demonstrable effect on neurotransmitters. One of Benedetti's studies,[6] for instance, found that a saline placebo not only reduces the symptoms of Parkinson's disease but can also increase the production of dopamine—the very neurotransmitter that Parkinson's robs from the brain.

Research has also suggested the existence of a *nocebo* effect—when a "dummy treatment," as placebos are sometimes called, offers both psychological and physiological consequences with *negative* results. (Nocebo, in Latin, means "I shall harm.") In one pioneering study,[7] fifteen patients receiving lumbar puncture, a procedure in which fluid is taken from the spine through a needle, were told to expect a headache afterward. In the end, seven of the fifteen patients reported having a headache. By contrast, when thirteen patients were not warned of this possible side effect, none of them reported experiencing a headache. Similarly, in a randomized controlled study, women who were given epidurals during labor were informed about the procedure using two styles of framing. One set was told, "We are going to give you a local anesthetic that will numb the area, and you will be comfortable during the procedure," while the other was warned, "You are going to feel a big beesting; this is the worst part of the procedure."[8] The women given the positive prompt reported significantly less pain than those who were offered the more negative setup, despite the fact that they both had the same procedure.

In addition to our expectations subconsciously leading us to better—or, in the case of the nocebo, worse—health, our interactions with doctors and health-care practitioners can also improve our sense of well-being. This is known generally as the

Hawthorne effect,[9] or the observer effect, in which people modify an aspect of their behavior in response to their awareness of being watched. In a medical context, this is expressed, as studies have shown, when a person feels that a doctor is particularly attentive, their health improves more quickly.

Ted Kaptchuk, a prominent professor at Harvard Medical School (as well as a former practicing acupuncturist) and director of Harvard's Program in Placebo Studies and the Therapeutic Encounter (PiPS) at Beth Israel Deaconess Medical Center, has received millions of dollars in grants from the National Institutes of Health (NIH) to study placebos and has published numerous articles about his research in prestigious medical journals.[10] In an effort to offer scientific evidence of this secondary placebo effect—that there are health benefits associated with a positive transaction between medical caregiver and patient—Kaptchuk designed a fascinating study.[11] In collaboration with gastroenterologists, Kaptchuk studied patients suffering from irritable bowel syndrome (IBS), a chronic gastrointestinal disorder accompanied by pain and constipation. They split 262 participants into three groups: a control group, who were told they were on a wait list for treatment; a group who received "sham" acupuncture, which, as I described in Chapter 5, entails using retractable needles or administering needles at non–acupuncture points, without much interaction with the practitioner; and, last, a group who received sham acupuncture along with pampering care— which meant patients were engaged in at least twenty minutes of conversation including empathetic and hopeful sentiments expressed by the practitioner such as "I know how difficult this is for you" and "This treatment has excellent results" while occasionally touching their hands and shoulders. To top it off, the practitioner was asked to spend at least twenty seconds lost in thoughtful silence—as if in quiet fascination with this particular medical dilemma—while they discussed the patient's care. It came as no surprise to Kaptchuk that the patients who experienced the greatest alleviation of symptoms were those who were attended to with great care.[12] But this study offering evidence of a "dose-dependent" response to placebo—in which the personal care was also one of the false remedies—made an impression on the medical community: bringing compassion and attentiveness into their practices was something that doctors could alter in practice realistically and immediately to achieve better outcomes.[13]

Erik Peper suggests that the results of Kaptchuk's study can help us better understand the dynamics at work in energy healing. "We are wired to interpret the world as dangerous or safe—mostly this is a nonverbal, energetic quality," he says. In any interaction between two people, he says, "[t]here is also the process of mirror neurons [which have been found to fire when a person observes the same action performed by another—thus the neurons "mirror" the behavior of the other, as though the observer were actually acting]. So when a healer is there and you are anxious—here comes the person who is secure and comfortable so you feel safe and you are already upping your healing potential. And then the healer does something and you believe they are doing something positive and you interpret you are feeling different in your body—and that resets your beliefs."[14]

Kaptchuk's finding is also a rebuke of the traditional approach to the placebo: you cannot factor the placebo effect out of the equation because you cannot isolate the emotions and impressions elicited in a medical transaction. You feel safe or you don't, and either way, this plays a role, at least to some degree, in the outcome. Even before I learned this lesson proffered by placebos, I had always been very clear with my staff at my acupuncture clinic about the atmosphere I want to foster. It is common sense that a compassionate and dependable environment will help a patient to improve, but I also believe a supportive feeling should encompass *all* interactions—not just between practitioner and patient but among everyone in the practice. This foundational belief of our clinic, I believe, has aided our success.

There is, however, some unsettling evidence that suggests placebos are not always as harmless or as minimally invasive as we might like to believe. Ian Harris, professor of orthopaedic surgery at the University of New South Wales and author of *Surgery, the Ultimate Placebo*,[15] posits that even surgical procedures can have a placebo effect. In his experience and research he has found that, in some cases, an operation is conducted more as a gesture of reassurance than a necessary intervention. "If you were to build the perfect placebo," he says, "it would be invasive, it would be costly, it would be set up in an environment that is high-tech and full of professionals, the person delivering it would be a very confident practitioner. These are all of the things that make surgery have such a strong placebo effect."[16] Whereas patients are influenced by such pageantry, Harris suggests, surgeons have a difficult time letting go of both long-standing tradition and an investment in their own success. "It's very difficult to tell [surgeons] the procedure they've been doing their whole career doesn't work,"[17] Harris says. He points to spine fusion surgery as one procedure that has failed, more often than not, to be truly effective. There have been several studies,[18] according to Harris, that have compared spine fusion surgery for certain painful degenerative conditions in the back to noninvasive programs such as physical therapy or cognitive behavioral therapy. These have unilaterally shown that patients who undergo surgery fare no better than if they were to do the cognitive behavioral or physical therapies. "And so there is a question mark over the effectiveness," Harris says. "Compare it to operations like a hip replacement surgery, where the success rate is extremely high, something like 95 percent, and the chance of ever having to have your hip operated on again is very low . . . Meanwhile, the failure rate for spine surgery is very high and there is a need to have [follow-up] spine surgery in up to 20 percent of cases after only two years."[19] Additionally, Harris pointed out that knee arthroscopy, in which a small incision is made in the knee and a camera is inserted to view the joints, is a surgery that has been studied in comparison to placebo groups, receiving sham surgeries, with no difference in the outcome for the two groups.[20]

Peper believes it is important to make a distinction between using active and passive placebos when looking at the placebo effect. Generally, active placebos cause mild side effects (such as pills with a low dose of caffeine that can cause an increased heart rate); passive placebos cause no side effects, as with, for example, a low-dose sugar pill. Peper's research has shown that active placebos can lead to different study outcomes because once people feel a side effect, regardless of whether it has a connection to a real medication, they start to believe they are getting better. "Many medications or surgical procedures can appear effective, and they may be," Peper explains. "However, many have never actually been compared to an active placebo, only to a passive placebo. Especially with psychiatric drugs or some of the pain meds, the effect you get may not be due to the active ingredient of the medication but to the placebo effect—the body sensations caused by the medication's side effects."[21] With arthroscopic knee surgery, Peper believes that an active placebo—meaning a "mock" knee surgery in which a patient is given local anesthesia and an incision is made but no actual surgery is performed—is necessary to be used in comparison to real surgery because the patient experiences some pain from the incision and this can lead the participant to believe he has recovered based on this "side effect" alone.[22] Critics have noted that placebos, particularly when an invasive procedure is needlessly endured to obtain study results, are deceptive and therefore not ethically administered. On the other hand, there is evidence that patients are perfectly willing to withstand being treated with placebos, and it doesn't affect the outcome if they're aware that it's a sham treatment. Kaptchuk once devised an experiment[23] in which he explicitly told the participants they would be receiving pills that were inert, explaining that placebos are often as effective as medicine—and still nearly 60 percent of the participants reported feeling better.[24]

In recent years, many groundbreaking studies on the placebo effect have been published, several of which suggest that the effectiveness of pain medications may be largely attributable to their value as placebos. A 2015 study[25] published in the journal *Pain* concluded that over the course of seventeen years, the effectiveness of pain medications in clinical trials has declined sharply. In 1996, drugs relieved pain 27 percent more than a placebo in trials, whereas by 2013 that gap had shrunk to 9 percent. Similar studies have been conducted on the use of Valium, and have found that the drug has no apparent effect on anxiety unless the person knows they have taken it.

Researchers are still seeking a coherent explanation as to *why* the placebo effect is so strong, and growing stronger. One theory draws on Kaptchuk's finding that the interaction between practitioner and patient creates its own placebo effect. Clinical trials in the US have grown longer and have included more participants in the nearly two decades between 1996 and 2013. In 1990, an average trial was four weeks long whereas by 2013, it was twelve weeks long; along the same lines, the average trial in 1990 included fifty people or fewer, but in 2013, trials included seven hundred participants, on average. As these trials have grown, researchers have added more personal elements to the process, such as hiring nurses to consult with the participants. (And it's likely no coincidence that, in an era where the standard of care has been diminished by stringent HMO and insurance policies, patients are starved for this kind of reassuring attention.) Another theory suggests that these trials have become more rigorously conducted and are simply revealing an outcome that was always there: painkillers or antidepressants or surgery may be less effective than we think.[26]

Still others assert that the placebo effect is not psychological and chemical in nature but rather sociological and energetic. In fact, Bill Bengston, who you may remember from his studies on mice with cancer in Chapter 4, offers a radically different hypothesis. Building on his resonant bonding theory—which suggests that an energetic bond created by the engagement between researcher and participant can extend outward to others within a "meaning field" (recall the control mice who were unexpectedly cured in Bengston's experiment when they came into contact with the healers taking part in the study)—he believes that the two groups (control and not) of placebo effect studies are becoming entangled, so that the real stimulus given to one group also affects the other.[27] In other words, the control groups of these trials are similar to the control mice in his experiments—they are recovering because they become part of the meaning field.

I'd journeyed down quite a rabbit hole researching placebos and yet still the question remained: How much of what I achieve with patients can be attributed to the placebo effect? Ultimately I came to believe that as with medication, acupuncture, and energy healing generally, it likely contains an element of placebo. In its broadest sense, the placebo effect is anything harmless that prompts our body to heal itself—whether that is a sugar pill or a friendly rapport with a doctor—a category that both acupuncture and healing can fall under. In coming to this conclusion, I also realized that the placebo is not our enemy. Instead of battling or denying or isolating the placebo effect, we should be embracing it. If it is *working* as part of the healing process, as increasingly seems to be the case, then why fear it?

Similar to Kaptchuk's description of the discrete threads that become braided in making up the placebo effect—our brains, our bodies, the method of placebo delivery, the physical environment, the manner of the doctor—I also believe that energy healing is an intertwining of a variety of elements that are not always quantifiable. For example, in acupuncture, the placebo effect may take place in combination with the electrical intervention spread via the fascia. Or it may enhance the energetic prompt of hands-on healing, which creates measurable resonance between the healer and the patient, resulting in a feeling of safety that opens the patient to information that shifts the body's healing mechanism. Ultimately, I came to see that compassion and belief are powerful antidotes—and should be harnessed in whatever form they come in.

YOU THE HEALER

Harnessing the Mind-Body Connection

In Chinese philosophy, there is a saying: *Where the mind goes, qi follows.* This exercise helps to use the placebo effect in the sense that it triggers our own mental self-healing mechanisms. By visualizing blockage in your field, you are directing your body's intelligence toward places where it is needed. I use it with patients who are suffering from chronic pain, and they are often surprised to find it brings them relief. It's based on the idea that dense or blocked energy in the personal energy field leads to pain and dysfunction. As we learned in Chapter 3, force does not move dense energy in the body—gentleness and love do. In this meditation, you'll learn to identify areas of your body that store pain and then disperse the resulting stagnation.

Body Scanning

Lie down in a place that feels comfortable, such as on your bed or on a yoga mat on the floor.

Spend a few minutes practicing the resonant breathing from Chapter 2, by gently breathing in for a count of six and then breathing out for a count of six.

Once your mind feels quiet, gently scan your body for areas of tension or discomfort.

As you identify areas of tension, place your attention on those areas, without judgment.

Allow the thoughts, feelings, and beliefs associated with this area of your body to simply be present, informing you of the root of your discomfort but not binding you to it.

When it feels right, find a memory that invokes a feeling of safety and warmth.

Take this energy and direct it to the area of tension.

Allow the warmth to gently release any density or struggle.

As you feel the area release, return your focus to your breath.

Continue with the body scan, stopping to dissipate tension in other parts of your body.

This should take about thirty minutes. Once you are done, lie still for a few more minutes and notice how your experience of your body has changed.

9

YOU THE HEALER

Madhu Anziani was twenty-three years old when he accidentally fell out of the second-story window of his house in San Francisco, California. His roommates heard his cries and found Anziani coiled in agony on the brick courtyard below. When Anziani arrived at UCSF Medical Center, he was wheeled into a thirteen-hour surgery to fuse together multiple vertebrae of his neck. His parents, who were in New York City caring for his grandmother, granted permission for the surgery—"[My] life depended on it," Anziani explains. His father and sister immediately flew back to San Francisco to find that Anziani had made it through the surgery but was now in a coma. Though his spinal cord hadn't been completely severed, it was so badly damaged that the doctors warned his family he would likely be paralyzed from the neck down.

"They were worried I'd be a tetraplegic, meaning all four limbs are paralyzed. The odds were not in my favor," explains Anziani.

"Luckily my injury was incomplete—it didn't entirely sever my spine. If you sever your spine, you're 99.99 percent not going to heal. With an incomplete spinal cord injury, there is potential, there is chance."[1]

That chance was the opening—the light still able to come through the cracks—Anziani seized upon. He had, in a way, been preparing for this. He was a student at the Institute for Holistic Health Studies program at San Francisco State University— where Erik Peper was one of his teachers—studying energy healing modalities with a focus on Reiki and sound healing. The program teaches a holistic awareness of illness and treatment, recognizing the interdependence of emotions, physiological processes, and environment, while also drawing on cultures around the world to understand a range of healing traditions.

Anziani's father and sister contacted Anziani's Reiki teacher within a day of their arrival, asking her to teach them about this practice, which originated in Japan in 1922 and uses a technique called "palm healing," more generally referred to as hands-on healing, that basically entails a practitioner channeling energy while gently placing his or her hands on a patient's head and torso. The Reiki teacher invited Anziani's sister and father to work with her for a day; she gave them both treatments in order to help them understand this healing therapy. She also taught them how to perform Reiki so that they could try it with Anziani too. Anziani's father, sister, and Reiki teacher practiced on Anziani every day while he was in the coma; they enlisted family and friends to visit, to talk to him, to pray for him.

When Anziani regained consciousness after eighteen days, he found that he couldn't speak. For a long while, he remained silent, watching as the others bustled about him. After a month, however, when he tried yet again to muster his voice, a sound came out—a very weak "ah" emerged. From then on, "what I knew to do was to make the 'ah' sound," he says. "I felt the vibration throughout my body, throughout my nervous system, going into my legs . . . [so] I would make the sound for five minutes at a time. I kept trying to increase the amount of time I could do it."[2] It gave him a feeling of "aliveness" in his body, as Anziani puts it, "and it was not subtle." This tone—now a protracted "aaaaaaah" chant—was calming. As Anziani got stronger and was able to expand the sounds he could vocalize, he began to recite a Sanskrit mantra, the first mantra he'd ever been taught: *Om mani padme hum.* "*Om*" symbolizes the speaker's impure body, speech, and mind; "*mani*," literally meaning "jewel," symbolizes a compassionate intention to become enlightened; "*padme*," meaning "lotus," symbolizes wisdom; the final syllable, "*hum*," suggests indivisibility.[3] This phrase is often etched on the outside of a prayer wheel—or it is written on paper and inserted into the prayer wheel—which is meant to be spun while chanting. Anziani, too, had a prayer wheel, and, although he was not able to spin it, his father would help him to reach out his hand and touch the wheel while chanting the mantra.

When he was in Dr. Peper's class at SFSU, Anziani had studied, as he describes it, "the power of our mind and the power of the placebo effect and the power of our words and the power of visualizing to create real results."[4] He also mentioned—and this came as a surprise to both of us—a guest speaker who had visited and been one of the most influential people in helping him to believe in energy healing: Hiroyuki Abe. "I saw him perform an instantaneous energy healing session on a woman," says Anziani. "She wasn't able to bend over and touch her toes, and, after about a minute of energy work [with Abe], she could do it."[5]

Anziani credits his knowledge of and confidence in energy healing as an essential part of his rehabilitation. The doctors were supportive, even amazed, by Anziani, as they noted that he was recovering more movement in a shorter amount of time than they'd expected. "One of my nurses called me 'the teacher,'" says Anziani, "because she'd seen the devotional healing happening around me and that I was doing for myself." But they remained understandably dubious about a full recovery. "There are many people with incomplete spinal cord injury who are in wheelchairs for the rest of their lives," Anziani points out. "So it is hard to know [what will happen]. The rehab program is about trying your best and seeing what you can get back . . . If you're lucky, you might be able to sit upright or maybe even stand on your feet for five minutes."[6] Still Anziani always held an image of himself walking out of the hospital in his mind's eye. When he confided this to one of the nurses, she gently told him not to have thoughts like that and encouraged him to focus instead on learning to adjust to his new life as a tetraplegic.

"Every time I was told that I would have to live a certain way, an adapted lifestyle, I didn't let it penetrate me," Anziani says. "I didn't let it be my belief system. I let it just be there. Of course, it was possible that I was going to be a disabled person. But I also knew that my thoughts are powerful, feelings are powerful, they generate energy and chemicals in your body. I knew that visualizing [myself walking] was a better option than some sort of a story of a disabled life. So I used my mind to transcend the

perceived reality and tap into the ocean of healing love that exists
in every moment. I let there be joy in my body because I know
the presence of joy and gratitude heal."[7]

After two and a half months, Anziani was able, with the
help of a walker, to leave the hospital on his own two feet. He
could only go fifteen to twenty feet before he needed to sit down
again—but he did walk out. A year later, he was mobile enough
to travel by plane from California to New York to see his family.
"That was a milestone for me," he says, "to be in the world, not
as a tetraplegic in a wheelchair, but as someone who could walk
into public spaces and blend in."

Though it is an astounding story, really the only one I have
ever heard like it, it is *not* a miracle. I say this because "miracle"
connotes mystery, and though there is an element of Anziani's
recovery that remains hidden even to him, there are also elements
that can be identified and practiced, albeit in less radical ways, in
our everyday lives.

What I find so fascinating—and inspiring—about Anziani is
how gracefully he navigated being the healer *and* patient, requir-
ing engagement and surrender. As the patient, Anziani was committed enough to keep making the effort (to exercise his voice,
his lungs, his body) despite the uphill battle he faced, and yet,
as the healer, he let go of his ego—and a sense of being able to
control his outcome. Crucially, Anziani accepted the possibility
that he might not walk again, but he allowed this to coexist with
the understanding that envisioning a different outcome brought
with it both pleasure and potential.

I think Anziani was able to accomplish such a feat because he understood that, at our core, we are whole and safe—this is the part of us that is connected to source. Safe, in this sense, does not mean protected from, as in Anziani's case, paralysis or, more broadly, illness or death; it means that we are all connected to a larger energy field that is both enlightened and altruistic—and willing to collaborate if we engage it. It is this part of ourselves—the aspect that is whole and safe—that good healers attempt to reconnect patients to by providing a prompt to the body's intelligence and ability to repair itself. Many healing modalities have the ability to urge the body toward health in this way: acupuncture, Reiki, shamanism, hands-on healing such as Bill Bengston tested in his lab, to name a few. But it is also possible to create this prompt for yourself.

The first step is to trust in your inherent ability to heal in a variety of ways. As I hope this book has shown, it is possible to document the process of self-healing in a wide variety of ways: scientific, spiritual, and experiential. Our greatest strength in healing, I believe, comes from an acceptance that our bodies—and spirits—are innately capable as opposed to vulnerable. When people get sick, they tend to blame themselves in overt and subtle ways, believing that they've somehow devised their own illnesses. But illness is not about weakness or blame; it's a natural call to bring our bodies back into coherence. Sometimes energy medicine can help to do this, and sometimes it can't, just as more generally, sometimes illness reverses and sometimes it doesn't. We will all become sick, and we will all die eventually; as I learned while working in hospice, dying is a transition, not an end, and, as a healer, it was my job to help those patients advance with as much fortitude and peace as possible. "Healing and curing aren't always synonymous. For some, healing may happen at the physical level immediately," writes Diane Goldner in her excellent book *Yes, You Can Heal: The Secret to Transforming Illness and Creating a Radiant Life.* "Sometimes it won't completely transfer to the physical plane—it might be about gaining a new perspective on life. It might even be about passing in a more free and conscious way. In any case, healing is about a state of being that is exciting and expansive."

And we can urge ourselves toward this expansive place, first by identifying where there is stagnation (specific steps for doing this can be found in the exercise at the end of Chapter 8) and altering our energy to call forth our essential vitality. The energy field is a template for the body; working with it creates change that then can affect our physical states.

Anziani, amazingly, was able to move his energy using the only method left available to him—sound. Master Kawakami, you will remember from Chapter 7, also sings during his healing sessions, in order to enter into a more receptive state as well as to allow his patients to become more open. He and Anziani are drawing from an idea passed down over history through many cultures—ancient Egyptians, Tibetan monks, Australian Aaorigines, Native American shamans, and Hindu healers among them—that have used chants and mantras and instruments such as singing bowls to restore the vibratory frequencies of the body and mind.

Sound occurs only when its vibration becomes a wave that hits the eardrum and is then recognized by our nerve centers. While it is self-evident that sound—chanting, chimes, the sonorous "ommmmm" intoned at the end of a yoga class—can make us feel more relaxed, the effects of sound are more than psychological; they are physiological: the vibrational energy of sound impacts our bodies on the cellular level and has the ability to lower heart rate variability and relax brain wave patterns. Studies have also shown that chanting certain mantras can stimulate the vagus nerve,[8] the longest cranial nerve in the body, which interfaces with the parasympathetic control of the heart, lungs, and digestive tract; appropriately, "vagus," in Latin, means "wanderer," as this nerve happens to do just that, winding all throughout the body to connect with various major organs. You might remember, too, this was the nerve Dr. Lagos suggested might be affected when I was treating others, triggering a rapid heartbeat and ultimately resulting in my tachycardia episodes. Singing and chanting, however, positively stimulate the activity of the vagus nerve, sending relaxing waves through the body and, as research has shown, increasing the production of oxytocin, sometimes referred to as "the love hormone," which conjures a sense of contentment.[9]

Vibrations are not only generated by sound, however; they can also be achieved with light and even human touch. It's possible to produce them within yourself by practicing resonant breathing (explained in the exercise at the end of Chapter 2), chanting, or singing. This works to move the energy within us because vibrations allow energy to travel in waves.

Yet Anziani did not simply chant himself into wellness. The healing process involves the act of affecting our energy and our energy fields, as well as a shift in our belief systems. Anziani was genuinely open to possibility; he did not have any limiting beliefs, or what Neale Donald Walsch would call a Sponsoring

Thought. The Sponsoring Thought is, you'll remember, a hidden yearning or a confining emotion—*I am so afraid I will not get better*—that is driving your behavior. (I have also seen patients whose yearning was attached to the attention that their illness has brought them; it is not uncommon to find a kind of solace in others caring for you, not to mention slowing the world down for a bit.) This can be difficult to address, and even more difficult to let go—few of us, myself included, are able to achieve the absolute openness of Abe or Kawakami or Anziani—but it *is* possible to recognize when fear or anger or shame are the primary generators of your actions. These feelings create obstacles to aligning with the whole version of yourself in order to more fully inhabit it. And I have found that change occurs when a patient allows for a liberating shift in mind-set, which often means addressing uncomfortable emotions and thought patterns head-on.

Emotions, as neuroscientific research has shown,[10] operate at a much higher speed than thoughts because they most often bypass the mind's linear reasoning process. As such, negative emotions—such as fear and anxiety—can make the heartbeat more erratic, signaling to the body that the nervous system is out of sync and initiating a cascade of 1,400 biochemical changes that have an array of effects on the body.[11]

The late Candace Pert, PhD, a neuroscientist, pharmacologist, and the first female chief at the National Institute for Mental Health, as the chief of brain biochemistry, became internationally recognized while only a graduate student at Johns Hopkins University for playing a key role in discovering the opiate receptor, the cellular binding site for endorphins, the body's natural painkillers, in the brain. Pert is also known, however, for becoming a lead proponent of Mind Body medicine—she preferred not to hyphenate the words to emphasize how closely the two are interlinked—and a forceful advocate for a more holistic approach to understanding health.

"I've come to believe that virtually all illness, if not psychosomatic in foundation, has a definite psychosomatic component," she wrote in her book *Molecules of Emotion: The Science Behind Mind-Body Medicine*.[12] Based on her research, Pert asserted that emotions play an essential role in disease. Receptors exist on every cell in the body, she explained, and when they become activated by our "molecules of emotion"—the neuropeptides (chemicals used by the brain to communicate with the body) that flood our systems—the receptor passes a charge into the cell, changing its electrical frequency as well as its chemistry. "Mind doesn't dominate body," Pert concluded, "it becomes body."

She also felt that, as our individual cells carry an electric charge, so, too, do our bodies. "We're vibrating like a tuning fork—we send out a vibration to other people. We broadcast and receive," Pert explained in an interview. "Feelings literally alter the electrical frequencies generated by our bodies, producing a nonverbal communication."

Which is not to say that you should never experience a negative emotion or encounter opposition within yourself; it is, of course, impossible to beat a perfect path toward emotional balance. In fact, at some point in the healing process you *will* encounter resistance. This can feel like a loss of faith or general depression or acute frustration. But don't give up: this is usually a resistance to the changes that are necessary to heal. Often patients going through this stage will project their emotion outward, not unlike the transference people can feel with their therapists. I've had some patients sob in the treatment room while others have become angry. Once, I treated a woman with acupuncture only to find a small pile of needles left on the table when I returned. She'd been so furious with the emotions that had come up with the movement of energy stimulated by the acupuncture, she'd pulled all of her needles out and stormed out of the treatment room while I'd been with another patient. When I called her to talk about what had happened, she had thankfully calmed down, and was conciliatory, but when I asked why she hadn't rung for me (all of my patients have a button they can press to summon me while they've got the needles in), she said, "I didn't want to see you." She had wanted instead to quietly escape the turmoil that her healing process was surfacing.

But the turmoil and resistance is the dynamic movement of energy necessary to effect change. So it is worth it to push through. To make it through this turbulent phase, it is important to remember that, as Kiran Trace taught me, you cannot move energy, or break up stagnation, with force or coercion. Try to use the same gentleness and support with yourself that you would expect, or hope for, from family members or practitioners. Similarly, gratitude, as Neale Donald Walsch instructs, creates movement in the energy field. "What you resist, persists," Walsch says. "But what you look at with gratitude ceases to have illusory form." Both are saying the same thing: to align with the energetic version of yourself, your blueprint, that is whole and free from suffering, you need to resonate with it. And to do so, you need to acknowledge, and trust, your own ingenuity as well as that of source. Anziani did just this when he "let there be joy in

[his] body," as he describes it, even as he was unable to move. He also facilitated this by using visualization, which is an incredibly useful tool for accessing a more positive feeling. It is important to remember too: you are never alone. The broader field is there for you to draw from and, once you have pushed past resistance and are able to coax yourself along, you will enter into a more productive exchange with the broader energy field, or source.

Though I believe we all possess the power to heal ourselves, it is also crucial to understand that, especially in an extreme case such as Anziani's, recovery is the result of a combination of interventions. Western medicine is thorough and profound, offering a powerful mode of healing that is utterly distinct from energy healing, which is why I'm a firm believer in integrative partnerships between medical doctors and energy medicine practitioners. (This kind of alliance has been institutionalized in such reputable places as Memorial Sloan Kettering Cancer Center, the Mayo Clinic, UCSF Medical Center, and Duke University School of Medicine, which have brought acupuncturists on staff in order to offer an integrative approach for their patients.)

Get advice, get help, and assemble the best team of practitioners you can—but also remember that *you* are ultimately your own best healer. What was startling to me about Anziani—able to stand out even amidst his miraculous recovery—was the fact that he, at the age of twenty-three, never gave away any of his own power. He truly understood the resources at his disposal, making appropriate use of everybody's skills, while maintaining conviction in his own beliefs—even as others, including those in positions of medical authority, tried to dissuade him. He demonstrated that, exercising faith and agency, it is possible to uncover an astounding healing capacity within us.

There is something excellently democratic about this, carrying within it an intrinsic, and crucial, check on the ego. As healers are ordinary people, each one brings their own individual character traits to their work. Some express their talents with dramatic flair—think of Kawakami with a skewer through his tongue—while others have more of a scientific bent, such as Bengston with his mice in the lab. In understanding that the healing profession is as varied as any other, it's also true that not all healers possess the same intentions and integrity. I've met dozens of accomplished healers in the course of my career who are engaged in committed and compassionate work. But I have also met others, albeit a small minority, who use their position to manipulate and deceive. It is always shocking to come across a person who has become so obscured to himself, or herself, it is no longer possible for them to differentiate their compulsive needs from their actions. Damaging therapeutic relations, of course, occur throughout medicine, but this can be particularly insidious in unlicensed medical realms, when practitioners are likelier to have had unorthodox training and are less likely to be held accountable. (A licensed medical practitioner hazards losing his license, and livelihood, if he crosses a line into unprofessional behavior.)

And although I have witnessed only a few infractions among other healers, I have seen enough red flags to consult with a forensic psychiatrist who focuses on maintaining boundaries in clinical practice. Dr. Thomas Gutheil, professor of psychiatry, cofounder of the Program in Psychiatry and Law at Beth Israel Deaconess Medical Center at Harvard Medical School, and author of the book *Preventing Boundary Violations in Clinical Practice*,[13] has seen professional abuses ranging from a healer convincing his patient not to get a second opinion to some who were abusing their power to sleep with vulnerable patients and another who was getting patients to run his errands.[14]

"Think of these people as a cult of one," Gutheil says.

Most of these detrimental relationships begin with the healer going on a charm offensive, creating both credibility and a sense of reliability, followed by a sense of emotional intimacy and, ultimately, dependence. Given the nature of the relationship—often with the patient feeling that the practitioner has some degree of authority over their well-being—patients are apt to feel vulnerable and lower their guard more quickly than usual. Confirmation bias, or the tendency to interpret new evidence as affirmation of existing beliefs or theories, also plays a critical role. Given the unusual intertwining of medical and spiritual beliefs of most healing practices, patients tend to believe the healer is uniquely placed to help them, leading them to ignore clues that might show fallibility or limitations.

I have also seen practitioners use their fee as a way of asserting a kind of dominance over the patient. When a healer charges an exorbitant fee, for example, patients are inclined to overvalue the service, to make the investment feel worthwhile. Paradoxically, I've also come across Svengali-like healers who charged no fee at all. This lulls patients into a false sense of security while the healer is able to solidify his or her "brand," and ultimately monetize their following.

A major warning sign for Gutheil is when a practitioner declares that they are the only one who can help. I am—as was Gutheil—hard-pressed to imagine a scenario in which this would ever be true. In a number of cases that Gutheil investigated, the doctor promised to be the patient's "everything," and the patient was elated to find someone who could—and would—take care of them in that way. The assumption, Gutheil explained, is that the therapy will solve not just the medical issues for which the patient is seeking help but all of life's difficulties.

"In theory, every physician [and practitioner] should get only two things from the patient," Gutheil succinctly explains. "[One] is their fee and the other is the satisfaction of doing the job well."[15] If a practitioner is using the therapeutic relationship to achieve more than this, there is a risk of the patient being exploited. Fortunately, unscrupulous practitioners are rare, and there is a simple way to protect yourself. As he lay in his hospital bed, Anziani used every tool at his disposal to prompt his body's own intelligence to restore order, and he never gave that power away. It was, I believe, the key to his recovery, because he understood that, at the most fundamental level, we are our own healers.

YOU THE HEALER

Self-Healing

Every day, we heal ourselves in ways that go unnoticed. That's because our bodies are designed to quietly restore homeostasis and return to a state of balance. When we overindulge, our digestive systems and organs of detoxification work overtime to offset any damage. When we catch viruses, our immune systems spring into action ready to fight. If we cut ourselves, our blood cells clump together to form a clot to stop the bleeding. It's easy to take these everyday miracles for granted, but they are a result of the body's innate intelligence and coherence. Energy medicine can give your body the information or prompt it needs to reorganize. This meditation brings together the exercises from earlier in the book, to boost your body's self-healing abilities.

- You can practice this exercise lying down or sitting comfortably with a straight spine.
- Start your meditation by opening to the universal energy field using the grounding and opening exercise from Chapter 3. Visualize a laser from your lower spine sinking deep into the earth. Allow yourself to feel heavier. Then imagine a ball of light, your own spiritual light, entering your body through the top of your head and flowing through you.
- To put your body in a receptive state, spend a few minutes practicing the resonant breathing from Chapter 2 by gently breathing in for a count of six and then breathing out for a count of six.
- As your mind relaxes, feel your body's vitality by using the experiencing energy exercise from Chapter 1.
- At this point I'm going to give you a choice. Over the

course of this book, we have learned a number of different techniques that help the body reorganize. Pick the one that feels appropriate and spend ten minutes doing it.

- To get out of your own way and let your body access the information it needs, use the rapid image cycling exercise from Chapter 4.
- For specific symptoms and to affect the energy channels, use the acupressure exercise from Chapter 5.
- For a general tune-up, use the chakra meditation from Chapter 6.
- To deepen your intuition by expanding your consciousness, use the circular breathing exercise from Chapter 7.
- To find areas of dense energy and dissipate them, use the body scanning exercise from Chapter 8.

- At some point during this exercise, you may feel resistance. It can take the form of intrusive thought of physical discomfort. There's no need to fight this resistance. Simply acknowledge it for what it is and feel the same compassion for yourself that you would for another person. Dr. Lagos, the psychologist from Chapter 2, gave me this breathing exercise to help change your heart rhythm in order to shift your energy. She tells me that the athletes she coaches use it to let go after a bad shot.
  - Five breaths (focusing on a negative emotion such as stress, anger, or disappointment on inhale and releasing it from the body on the exhale)

- • Five breaths to clear the mind (focusing on the feeling
    of the inhale and exhale)
  - • Five breaths to boost the heart (focusing on a positive
    emotion such as love, gratitude, or serenity on the
    inhale and letting go of the negative on the exhale)
- As you feel your body's energy, allow the sense of vitality
  to bring you joy and say thank you. Expressing gratitude
  is one way of aligning yourself with the future version of
  yourself that you are envisaging.
- When you are ready, get up and notice any changes in
  your body.

10

LET THERE BE LIGHT

On my last day with Hiroyuki Abe in Japan, I accompanied him to his student's clinic outside of Kobe, where he occasionally holds healing sessions. After several hours in a small classroom observing Abe and several of his students as they treated patients, we started to pack up to leave. We were on our way out the door to go to the shabu-shabu restaurant for dinner—the dinner, in fact, where Abe would, by shaking two fingers at my chest, put my heart back into normal rhythm during my tachycardia episode. At this moment, however, Abe stopped us from walking out of the classroom and turned to me, asking me through his translator if I'd like him to attune me to his energy and open my chakras, the very ceremony he performs for his apprentices when they begin working with him. I could tell from the reaction among his students that this was an unusual offer. I felt it was a profound honor and accepted.

Abe motioned for me to sit down in front of him. I did so and closed my eyes. I heard Abe snapping his fingers behind me, and I could feel the motion of his hands along the back of my head and down my spine, though he wasn't actually touching me. Almost immediately, I saw a white light, and then bright colors appeared, swirling within the light. My body began to buzz with an electric energy. I felt an uneasy sense of anticipation, an exaggerated version of the feeling I get when I'm on a plane about to take off. The colors continued to spiral, like a kaleidoscope, and I took deep breaths, trying to calm down. (Later, when I watched a video that my husband recorded as this was happening, I would see that Abe pushed both his hands downward, as if he were trying to resist the rising energy, bringing it down to a more comfortable level, with an effortful grimace.) I felt dizzy, exhilarated, and somewhat overwhelmed. Needing to come back to reality, I opened my eyes.

Something had changed. The room was now filled with a warmer, encompassing light. I couldn't help but think of the light my mother had once described seeing as she was being resuscitated on a gurney in the hospital when she was near death. This light, too, felt embracing. My mother had described that moment as the safest she had ever felt in her life. Abe's students now seemed to be shining, bathed in this radiant light. It felt as if I were seeing everyone as pure energy. For the first time, I understood, in as visceral and complete a way as I ever had, that our vitality, our animating force, the very thing that makes us vibrant individuals, is also, paradoxically, what connects us. We all share in this light, this energy. It's expansive; it communicates with us, and it *is* essentially who we are. I was seeing, I felt, our true nature.

In Chinese philosophy, everything in the world has an opposite, and it is this way for a reason. "Yin-yang" is literally translated as "dark-bright"; it is meant to describe how contrary forces can be complementary and interconnected. Opposites such as darkness and light, or energy and matter, as Chinese philosophy posits, are physical representations of duality in nature and are considered a manifestation of our oneness—and the Tao. As Neale Donald Walsch understands it: every living being is essentially source having a physical experience, and it is in this way that source is able to experience duality—the light and the dark.

I have come to believe that light—as well as the duality that these philosophic and spiritual beliefs describe—may play a role in the healing process. The human body does actually, quite literally, emit light in very small quantities. In fact, all living creatures emit very weak light. It is visible, though not to the human eye. In 2009, researchers in Japan, using a highly sensitive imaging system with a "cryogenic charge-coupled device (CCD) camera," captured images of the biophoton emission—particles of light produced by a biological system—of the human body.[1] They studied five healthy males in their twenties, who stood bare-chested in front of CCD cameras in complete darkness for twenty minutes every three hours, from ten a.m. to ten p.m., three days in a row. The images showed that, as the researchers wrote in their published findings, "the human body directly and rhythmically emits light." The glow of the men's bodies was at its lowest point at ten a.m. and its peak at four p.m., suggesting that this emission is linked to the body clock. The researchers concluded that these diurnal changes might be connected to energy metabolism fluctuations.

I am not suggesting that Abe unleashed an ability in me to see the ultra-weak biophoton emissions of others—what I experienced, I believe, is not something that can be pinned down by science—but I do think this research has relevance as we consider how we can harness energy to heal one another.

There is an interesting precedent to the findings of the Japanese researchers. They were building on the work of Fritz-Albert Popp, a German biophysicist, who, in the 1970s, offered the first extensive physical analysis of biophotons. Popp was also the first person to speculate that the human body produces very weak biophoton emissions and that they follow particular biorhythms of the body and the world—theories that, we now know, were later corroborated.

Perhaps more crucially, however, Popp deduced that our biophoton emissions might offer information about our health. Early on, Popp found that the molecule benzo[a]pyrene, a cancer-producing molecule, absorbed ultraviolet (UV) light but then re-emitted it at a completely different frequency—what Popp termed a "light scrambler." By contrast, the molecule benzo[e]pyrene, which is harmless to humans, allowed UV light to pass through it without any changes.[2] Fascinated by this difference, he went on to investigate the effect of UV light on other compounds, some cancer-causing and some not. In every instance, the carcinogenic substances absorbed the UV light and then scrambled the frequency. Popp also observed that the carcinogenic compounds consistently reacted to the UV light at a specific frequency: 380 nanometers (nm). Separately, in a process called photo repair, if UV light is directed at a cell so that 99 percent of it, including its DNA, is destroyed, the damage can be nearly repaired in a single day by illuminating the cell with light at a particular frequency—that frequency, Popp discovered, is also 380 nm.[3] This startling coincidence led Popp to conclude that cancer occurred in humans when carcinogens rendered photo repair impossible. He suggested that the photon emission of a healthy human is coherent, following the biorhythm he observed, whereas the photon emission of seriously ill people, such as those with cancer, loses its diurnal rhythm.

Popp subsequently studied light in DNA samples—using ethidium bromide, which inserts itself into the spaces between the base pairs of the double helix, to cause the DNA to unwind—and found that the more the DNA unraveled, the greater the intensity of light. He came to believe that DNA was the originating source of biophotons, and that it acted like a tuning fork in the body, striking a particular frequency that, in turn, provoked certain molecules to follow.[4]

Popp and his colleagues later performed a series of experiments, observing light emissions among fleas and fish, and found that they sucked up the light emitted from each other—an action that Popp termed "photon sucking."[5] He speculated that this might be a way of exchanging information—and could provide an explanation for some of the abiding mysteries of the animal kingdom, such as how schools of fish or flocks of birds fall into perfect and instantaneous coordination. For humans, he felt, there was this possibility: if we could take in the photons of others, we might be able to use this information to correct our own light if it is amiss.

Like sound, light is a vibration on the electromagnetic spectrum—the only difference between them being frequency.

Our bodies largely interpret frequencies unconsciously, and we do so more often than we likely realize. Various colors, for example, are simply different frequencies of light, which our brains interpret as a spectrum of colors. The same is true for how we decipher sensations of hot or cold or pain or pleasure; these are all frequencies that we filter and interpret. I have come to believe that specific vibrations—whether from light or sound—make up the information that is transferred from one person to another in energy healing.

The key to effectively exchanging this information—whereby one person is able to subtly shift the frequency or vibration of another—is resonance. This occurs, broadly speaking, when there is an exchange of energy between two systems. As I discovered in my work with Dr. Leah Lagos, when I am healing, I achieve internal resonance in which my heart and brain waves synchronize, creating calming signals that reverberate throughout my autonomic nervous system. This, in turn, allows me to both open to healing energy as well as more freely offer it to my patients. As Dr. Erik Peper explained, the phenomenon of mirror neurons—which have been found to fire when a person perceives another's actions as if they were actually performing that act—allows patients to follow my lead. In this sense, when I am able to synchronize my breathing and heart waves, creating a sense of calm, the patient, too, is able to do this; it is through this process that we come into resonance with each other. As I described in Chapter 2, Dr. Bill Bengston and his colleagues devised an experiment to record the physiological effects that occur when a healer and patient go into resonance. They found that even when the healer and patient were separated, in rooms thirty-five feet apart from each other, the healer's brain wave, initially stronger and more frequent, eventually synchronized with the patient—in other words, they achieved resonance.

The feeling I experience when I make this connection in a healing session is peaceful; it is a sense of limitlessness that I do not experience in any other part of my life. I once asked Bill Bengston to describe healing energy to me. I was curious to hear his explanation because it is, ultimately, an emotional response, and he is predominantly a technical, detail-oriented person. He has conducted some of the most granular research on healing I have seen. This is the man, after all, who has brought every aspect of his encounters with healing into the lab—from hands-on healing of mice to "charging" cotton with energy to sound recordings of him charging cotton in order to study its genomic effect on cancer. His studies are rigorous, and his lab work is meticulous. Bengston, himself, is perhaps the biggest skeptic I've met among healers.

Yet his answer to my question was this: "Healing is love."

This love comes from source energy. It has intelligence. It springs from the universal field as a movement that both flows through us and emanates from us. It is compassion and the recognition of our oneness. It allows for possibility. As healers we draw from this unconditional place—from the Tao—to help a patient release an interference or blockage that has interrupted the energetic flow in the body.

We are all capable of creating this connection. Healers are simply conduits. I have learned to open my body and mind to allow this to happen. All the healers in this book have learned to do this, though they've each created their own method of opening up to the energy. Bill Bengston distracts himself with cycling in order to surrender his ego; the naturopath Carla Kreft, who worked with me at Yinova, visualizes light streaming through her patients; Hiroyuki Abe communicates with the Shinto goddess of mercy while snapping his fingers and tapping certain points on the body; Master Mitsumasa Kawakami meditates on past lives and sings in piercing tones; Madhu Anziani used the only sound he could make to chant while lying paralyzed in his hospital bed. When Bill Bengston teaches his healing course, the first thing he does is hand a card to everyone in the class. It has two instructions: No ritual. Have fun. The point being that every one of us will have our own approach. Ritual will ultimately lead you astray; healing is a dynamic—and therefore ever-shifting—process.

"The light without any blocks is just pure flow," Kiran Trace said when I told her of my experience in the clinic with Abe. "This is how effortless awareness really is. [We are always] absorbing energy from this space . . . If you follow that flow deeper and deeper, it brings in clarity and information and eventually you will get to a vast, pure, empty spaciousness. [On one side of this,] energy moves into form but on the other, there is not just silence, there is love, and then there is pure radiant light."[6]

When I began writing this book, I was in search of tangible evidence that energy healing exists. I wanted to provide a systematic explanation—to myself and to my patients—for what I felt in my hands and tingling down my spine. I wanted to know what it was that I was offering. Throughout, I came across a seemingly endless line of fascinating people and conceivable explanations drawing on a variety of disciplines—philosophical, scientific, spiritual. And yet ultimately I have learned that though we can all experience it, we will never be able to fully describe it.

The Tao that can be spoken is not the eternal Tao.

YOU THE HEALER

Healing Others

As I hope I have made clear by now, an energy healer is essentially a conduit for energy—running through the body in the form of a vibration or wave—as opposed to someone who has been blessed or touched in an unusual way. Though some people are more attuned to their ability to heal than others, everyone has this ability within them. This exercise will help you use the information in this book, as well as incorporate the exercises you've been practicing along the way, to discover your potential as a healer. It's based on my own experience combined with what I learned from the energy healers and scientists that I met while writing this book. It's a safe way to deliver healing information to other people, and you can use it to help family and friends. It won't make you into an energy healer overnight, but if you practice you'll improve and you'll begin to create your own process. This is a short routine that will put your body into the internal resonance necessary to allow you to transmit information from your own energy field to someone else's field. The aim is to put both the healer and healee in a state where information transfer is possible. That doesn't require a fancy technique or precise ritual. It's more a state of being that recognizes our connection with source and the connection between you and the person you are aiming to help.

This doesn't replace conventional medical care, and it's important to communicate that to the healee. Do not encourage them to stop any current medications or in any other way give advice better suited to a medical professional.

1. Create a safe space.

See the healee as an expression of source energy and feel your connection to them. Respect them by committing to keep any information they reveal confidential and by dropping any judgments you may have of them.

2. Ask the healee to lie down and ensure that they are comfortable.

Being comfortable helps the patient to be receptive. A massage table is ideal for this because the height allows you, the healer, to stand comfortably and in a way that energy can flow through you. But truthfully you can transmit this energy with the patient in any position, including sitting or standing.

3. Ground and open to source.

Stand next to the patient and take a moment to get centered before you begin the session. Stand with your feet shoulder-width apart and bend your knees slightly, feeling your feet on the floor. Drawing on the grounding and opening exercise from Chapter 3, tilt your pelvis forward slightly and straighten your spine.

Imagine a cord of energy, like a laser beam, traveling from the base of your spine deep into the earth. Notice whether you feel heavier and more grounded. Imagine a ball of bright light above you and then visualize that light entering your body through the top of your head. Feel the light filling your body, extending through your trunk and into your limbs.

4. Distract your mind to allow energy to flow.

To do this, you can use the rapid image cycling from Chapter 4, which is a technique that takes some practice. Alternatively, simply distract your mind. I often look out of the window or even chat with the patient. That's my way of avoiding having my ego attached to the outcome of the healing and so making myself receptive.

5. Energize your hands.

Practice the experiencing energy exercise from Chapter 1 by placing your hands in front of you, with your palms facing each other and allowing them to move backward and forward focusing on the change in sensation. Once you feel energy flowing, hold your hands over the patient's and allow them to move as if guided by an outside force.

6. Allow energy to flow.

Don't force this to happen. Remember that source energy runs through you at all times and doesn't need to be invoked. I sometimes find my body moves of its own accord when the energy starts flowing. It's as if it lines me up so it can flow smoothly.

7. Disconnect from the patient.

Imagine the healee surrounded by white light and then visualize your own body surrounded by the light too. In doing this you are sending the message that although you are connected by source, you are both individuals with free will.

ACKNOWLEDGMENTS

My patients have taught me a great deal. I'm grateful to them for trusting me with their health care and for sharing their stories with me.

Speaking of stories, Nell Casey helped me to tell this one. A writer and editor, Nell helped me weave the strands of my own experience with the stories of the healers I met and the scientific research that supports their work. Nell and I were lucky enough to collaborate with researcher Michael Lowell, a meticulous fact-checker, who read countless books and hundreds of articles and interviewed dozens of people while working on this project. Kristina Grish worked on the original concept for this book and contributed to its structure. I'm grateful to them for all their hard work and talent.

Laura Nolan is my literary agent and has guided me wisely. She played an important role in shaping this book, and I'm thankful for her patience and support.

I jumped at the chance to be published by HarperCollins, and I appreciate their faith in this project. Harper Wave has published some of my favorite health books, and I couldn't wish for a better home as an author. The Harper Wave team, led by Karen Rinaldi, are talented and knowledgeable, and it's good to have them in my corner. Our editor, Julie Will, offered clarity and insight, and I appreciate her experience and the hard work that went into transforming our manuscript into this book.

There were times when I became consumed by this journey, and I'm thankful that my family was patient with me. My husband, Noah, and my daughter, Emma, work alongside me at Yinova (Noah runs the clinic and Emma runs the marketing department), and they both increased their own workloads so I could focus on this book. More than that, they were a source of inspiration, encouragement, and hugs. Louie, our dog, sat on my knee, keeping me company while I wrote. I'm grateful to all three of them.

From its humble beginnings, Yinova is now a large practice. So big, in fact, that I can't list all my colleagues by name, but they know that they are in my heart. I love working with a gifted team of practitioners and support staff to create a healing environment. I do want to give a special shout-out to Liz Henning, our COO, who is the most organized person I know and ran the business when I was writing this book. My assistant, Hemaalya Omrao, also deserves credit for lovingly keeping me on track.

Several academics and scientists contributed to this book. I'd like to thank Dr. Jeremy Pulsifer, who teaches physics to acupuncturists and is himself an accomplished practitioner of Chinese medicine, for his help identifying research relevant to our work. Dr. Bill Bengston, Dr. Erik Peper, Dr. Leah Lagos, Brenda J. Dunne, and Dr. Roger Nelson all patiently explained their work to us and were generous with their time and research.

In Japan, I was helped by a small army of translators, each of whom brought their own personality to the work. Kuzuhara

Kaori is a dainty woman with a tinkling laugh. Her grasp of English idiom was a marvel to me, and her humor and local knowledge made our trip to Kyoto, with Hiroyuki Abe, very special. Katsunori Kojima is a baseball announcer from Tokyo who lived in the USA while working as a translator for Tsuyoshi Shinjo when he played baseball for the New York Mets and later the San Francisco Giants. He flew to Kobe to translate my interview with Hiroyuki Abe, and his experience was evident when he was able to translate complex concepts while remaining neutral. We met up with him again in Tokyo, where he extended the hand of friendship, taking us to meet his parents and joining us for meals. Kojima was assisted by Sakiko Matsumoto, who provided backup translation for some interviews because of the esoteric nature of the subject matter. Takayuki Kawamoto was our translator in Fukuoka. He brought humor and warmth to the project and was a great help in understanding Master Kawakami's work. He was at times assisted by Erika Ashima, whose wry humor was very much appreciated. All of them took their work very seriously and made a huge contribution to this book.

I met many talented healers on this journey, and not all of them were featured in this book, but every one taught me something, and I'm grateful to them all for allowing me to observe their work and learn from them.

NOTES

Chapter 1: At My Fingertips

1. W. Beere, *Doing and Being: An Interpretation of Aristotle's Metaphysics Theta* (Oxford, UK: Oxford University Press, 2009), 160.
2. "The Higgs boson," CERN, accessed September 2017, https://home.cern/topics/higgs-boson.
3. O. J. Pike et al., "A Photon–Photon Collider in a Vacuum Hohlraum," *Nature Photonics* 8 (2014): 434–36.
4. Ibid.
5. A. El-Osta et al., "Transient High Glucose Causes Persistent Epigenetic Changes and Altered Gene Expression During Subsequent Normoglycemia," *Journal of Experimental Medicine* 205, no. 10 (2008): 2409–17.
6. Third Ch'an Patriarch Chien-chih Seng-ts'an, "Hsin-hsin Ming," Faith Mind Inscription, http://www.sacred-texts.com/bud/zen/fm/fm.htm.
7. Ibid.
8. Clyde Hughes, "Einstein Wrong about 'Spooky Action at a Distance,'" Newsmax, https://www.newsmax.com/thewire/albert-einstein-spooky-action-at-a-distance/2018/05/10/id/859478/.
9. Sir Isaac Newton, *Principia: The Mathematical Principles of Natural Philosophy* (New York: Geo. P. Putnam, 1850), https://books.google.com/books/about/Newton_s_Principia.html?id=N-hHAQAAMAAJ&printsec=frontcover&source=kp_read_button#v=onepage&q&f=true.

Chapter 2: The Science of Connection

1. Sir Isaac Newton, *Principia: The Mathematical Principles of Natural Philosophy* (New York: Geo. P. Putnam, 1850).
2. J. Z. Buchwald, *The Creation of Scientific Effects: Heinrich Hertz and*

Electric Waves (Chicago: University of Chicago Press, 1994); I. Adawi, "Centennial of Hertz' Radio Waves," *American Journal of Physics* 57 (1989): 125–27.

3. Max Planck, "Das Wesen der Materie" [The Nature of Matter] (speech in Florence, Italy, 1944) from *Archiv zur Geschichte der Max-Planck-Gesellschaft,* Abt. Va, Rep. 11 Planck, Nr. 1797).

4. L. McTaggart, *The Field: The Quest for the Secret Force of the Universe* (New York: HarperCollins Publishers, 2008), 32.

5. Ibid., 33.

6. M. Lincoln and A. Wasser, "Spontaneous Creation of the Universe Ex Nihilo," *Physics of the Dark Universe* 2, no. 4 (2013): 195–99.

7. L. McTaggart, *The Field: The Quest for the Secret Force of the Universe* (New York: HarperCollins Publishers, 2008), 19.

8. Ibid.

9. Ibid., 20.

10. Ibid., 23.

11. H. Puthoff, "Everything for Nothing," *New Scientist* (July 28, 1990): 52–55.

12. H. Puthoff, "The Energetic Vacuum: Implications for Energy Research," *Speculations in Science and Technology* 13 (1990): 247–57.

13. H. S. Burr, C. T. Lane, and L. F. Nims, "A Vacuum Tube Microvoltmeter for the Measurement of Bioelectric Phenomena," *Yale Journal of Biology and Medicine* 10 (1936): 65–76.

14. H. Burr, *The Fields of Life* (New York: Ballantine, 1972).

15. H. S. Burr, C. T. Lane, and L. F. Nims, "A Vacuum Tube Microvoltmeter for the Measurement of Bioelectric Phenomena," *Yale Journal of Biology and Medicine* 10 (1936): 65–76.

16. H. Burr, *The Fields of Life* (New York: Ballantine, 1972), 12–13.

17. W. Thomas, *The Force Is with Us: The Higher Consciousness That Science Refuses to Accept* (Wheaton, IL: Quest Books, 2009), 46, Kindle.

18. M. Goldman, A. Goldman, and R. S. Sigmond, "The Corona Discharge, Its Properties and Specific Uses," *Pure and Applied Chemistry* 57, no. 9 (1985): 1353–62.

19. W. Thomas, *The Force Is with Us: The Higher Consciousness That Science Refuses to Accept* (Wheaton, IL: Quest Books, 2009), 46, Kindle.

20. J. Hubacher, "The Phantom Leaf Effect: A Replication, Part 1," *Journal of Alternative and Complementary Medicine* 21, no. 2 (2015): 83–90.

21. P. Brook, "Aura Portraits Make Good Art, Bad Science," Wired.com, December 25, 2011, https://www.wired.com/2011/02/aura-portraits/.

22. T. Moss, "Puzzles and Promises," *Osteopathic Physician* (February 1976), 30–37.

23. H. Burr, *The Fields of Life* (New York: Ballantine, 1972).

24. R. O. Becker and G. Selden, *The Body Electric* (New York: Morrow, 1985): 73–74.

25. Ibid.

26. Leah Lagos, in discussion with the author, September 2017, New York.

27. www.heartmath.org.

28. L. Song, G. Schwartz, and L. Russek, "Heart-Focused Attention and Heart-Brain Synchronization: Energetic and Physiological Mechanisms," *Journal of Alternative and Complementary Medicine* 4, no. 5 (1998): 44–52, 54–60, 62.

29. G. E. Schwartz, *The Energy Healing Experiments: Science Reveals Our Natural Power to Heal* (New York: Astria Books, 2007), 78.

30. Leah Lagos, in discussion with the author, September 2017, New York.

31. P. M. Lehrer and R. Gevirtz, "Heart Rate Variability Biofeedback: How and Why Does It Work?" *Frontiers in Psychology* 5 (2014): 756.

32. Leah Lagos, in discussion with the author, September 2017, New York.

33. Ibid.

34. Ibid.

35. Ibid.

36. G. E. Schwartz, *The Energy Healing Experiments: Science Reveals Our Natural Power to Heal* (New York: Astria Books, 2007), 81.

37. Ibid., 87.

38. www.heartmath.org.

39. T. D. Duane and T. Behrendt, "Extrasensory Electroencephalographic Induction Between Identical Twins," *Science* 150, no. 3694 (1965): 3367.

40. L. Hendricks, W. F. Bengston, and J. Gunkelman, "The Healing Connection: EEG Harmonics, Entrainment and Schumann's Resonances," *Journal of Scientific Exploration* 25, no. 3 (1965): 419–30.

41. L. Hendricks W. Bengston, and J. Gunkleman, "The Healing Connection: EEG Harmonics, Entrainment, and Schumann's Resonances." *Journal of Scientific Exploration* 24, no. 4 (2010): 655–66.

42. B. J. Dunne, R. D. Nelson, and R. G. Jahn, "Operator-Related Anomalies in a Random Mechanical Cascade," *Journal of Scientific Exploration* 2, no. 2 (1988): 155–79.

43. Brenda Dunne, in discussion with the author, October 2017.

44. Ibid.

45. Ibid.

46. "Mind Over Matter," *The New York Times*, accessed May 1, 2017, https://www.nytimes.com/2003/03/09/nyregion/mind-over-matter.html.

47. Brenda Dunne, in discussion with the author, October 2017.

48. "The Global Consciousness Project Meaningful Correlations in Random Data," The Global Consciousness Project, accessed May 1, 2017, http://noosphere.princeton.edu./

49. Roger Nelson, in discussion with the author, January 2018.

50. "Trump Inauguration," The Global Consciousness Project, accessed May 1, 2017, http://teilhard.global-mind.org/events/trump.inaug.html; "Haiti Earthquake," The Global Consciousness Project, accessed May 1, 2017, http://teilhard.global-mind.org/haiti.quake.html.

51. Roger Nelson, in discussion with the author, January 2018.

52. B. J. Dunne and R. G. Jahn, "Experiments in Remote Human/Machine Interaction," *Journal of Scientific Exploration* 6 (1992): 311–32.

53. R. D. Nelson, "Anomolous Structure in GCP Data: A Focus on New Years," Global Consciousness Project, Princeton.

54. Roger Nelson, in discussion with the author, January 2018.

55. Ibid.

56. Ibid.

Chapter 3: What's God Got to Do With It?

1. B. Greyson, "Varieties of Near-Death Experience," *Psychiatry* 56, no. 4 (1993): 390–99.

2. Burton Watson, *Lao Tzu: Tao Te Ching* (Indianapolis: Hackett Publishing Company Inc., 1993).

3. N. D. Walsch, *Conversations with God* (New York: Penguin Group, 2005).

4. Ibid., 11.

5. Ibid.

6. Neale Donald Walsch, in discussion with the author, July 2017.

7. Ibid.

8. Ibid.

9. N. D. Walsch, *Conversations with God* (New York: Penguin Group, 2005), 91–92.

10. Ibid., 23.

11. Ibid., 38.

12. Ibid., 165.

13. Neale Donald Walsch, in discussion with the author, July 2017.

14. N. D. Walsch, *Conversations with God* (New York: Penguin Group, 2005).

15. Ibid., 165.

16. Kiran Trace, in discussion with the author, July 2017, New York.

17. Ibid.

18. Kiran Trace, *Tools for Sanity: Peace, Freedom and Fulfillment in Every Moment* (Mystic Girl in the City, 2013), 28, Kindle.

19. Kiran Trace, *Tools for Sanity: Peace, Freedom and Fulfillment in Every Moment* (Mystic Girl in the City, 2013), Kindle.

20. Ibid., 28.

21. Kiran Trace, in discussion with the author, July 2017, New York.

22. Kiran Trace, *Tools for Sanity: Peace, Freedom and Fulfillment in Every Moment* (Mystic Girl in the City, 2013), 893, Kindle.

23. Ibid., 897.

24. "Study Reveals Substantial Evidence of Holographic Universe," University of Southampton, https://www.southampton.ac.uk/news/2017/01/holographic-universe.page.

25. Ibid.

26. S. W. Hawking and T. Hertog, "A Smooth Exit From Eternal Inflation?" *Journal of High Energy Physics* 147 (2018).

27. N. Afshordi et al., "From Planck Data to Planck Era: Observational Tests of Holographic Cosmology," *Physical Review Letters* 118 (2017).

28. A. Beall, "Theory Claims to Offer the First 'Evidence' Our Universe Is a Hologram," *Wired*, http://www.wired.co.uk/article/our-universe-is-a-hologram.

29. S. W. Hawking and T. Hertog, "A Smooth Exit from Eternal Inflation?" *Journal of High Energy Physics* 147 (2018).

30. Ibid.

31. S. Cosier, "Could Memory Traces Exist in Cell Bodies?" *Scientific American*, 2015, https://www.scientificamerican.com/article/could-memory-traces-exist-in-cell-bodies/.

Chapter 4: Into the Lab

1. "SSE Conferences," The Society for Scientific Exploration, accessed May 1, 2017, https://www.scientificexploration.org/2017-conference.

2. W. Bengston and S. Fraser, *The Energy Cure: Unraveling the Mystery of Hands-On Healing* (Louisville, CO: Sounds True, Inc., 2005).

3. Ibid.

4. Ibid.

5. Ibid.

6. Ibid.

7. Ibid.

8. Ibid.

9. William Bengston, in discussion with the author, June 2017.

10. W. Bengston and S. Fraser, *The Energy Cure: Unraveling the Mystery of Hands-On Healing* (Louisville, CO: Sounds True, Inc., 2005).

11. D. Krinsley and T. Takahashi, "Surface Textures of Sand Grains: An Application of Electron Microscopy," *Science* 135 (1962): 923–25.

12. D. Krinsley and W. Wellendorf, "Wind Velocities Determined from the Surface Textures of Sand Grains," *Nature* 283 (1980): 372–73.

13. W. Bengston and S. Fraser, *The Energy Cure: Unraveling the Mystery of Hands-On Healing* (Louisville, CO: Sounds True, Inc., 2005).

14. Ibid., 80.

15. Ibid., 81.

16. Ibid., 176.

17. William Bengston, in discussion with the author, June 2017.

18. W. Bengston and S. Fraser, *The Energy Cure: Unraveling the Mystery of Hands-On Healing* (Louisville, CO: Sounds True, Inc., 2005), 159.

19. W. F. Bengston and D. Krinsley, "The Effect of the 'Laying On of Hands' on Transplanted Breast Cancer in Mice," *Journal of Scientific Exploration* 14 (2000): 353–64.

20. W. Bengston and S. Fraser, *The Energy Cure: Unraveling the Mystery of Hands-On Healing* (Louisville, CO: Sounds True, Inc., 2005).

21. W. F. Bengston and M. Moga, "Resonance, Placebo Effects, and Type II Errors: Some Implications from Healing Research for Experimental Methods," *Journal of Scientific Exploration* 13, no. 3 (2007): 317–27.

22. Imants Barušs, "Beyond Scientific Materialism Toward a Transcendent Theory of Consciousness," *Journal of Consciousness Studies* 17 (2010): 213–31.

23. W. Bengston and S. Fraser, *The Energy Cure: Unraveling the Mystery of Hands-On Healing* (Louisville, CO: Sounds True, Inc., 2005).

24. William Bengston, in discussion with the author, June 2017.

25. R. Sheldrake, *A New Science of Life: The Hypothesis of Formative*

Causation (London: Blond and Briggs, 1981); R. Sheldrake, *The Presence of the Past: Morphic Resonance and the Habits of Nature* (London: Icon Books Ltd., 2011).

26. Ibid.
27. William Bengston, in discussion with the author, June 2017.
28. W. F. Bengston and S. Fraser, *The Energy Cure: Unraveling the Mystery of Hands-On Healing* (Louisville, CO: Sounds True, Inc., 2005).
29. Ibid., 60.
30. William Bengston, in discussion with the author, June 2017.
31. Ibid.
32. Ibid.
33. Ibid.
34. William Bengston, in discussion with the author, June 2017.
35. W. F. Bengston, "Commentary: A Method Used to Train Skeptical Volunteers to Heal in an Experimental Setting," *Journal of Complementary and Alternative Medicine* 13, no. 3 (2007): 329–31.

Chapter 5: Moving the Needle

1. Luigi Galvani (1737–1798). *De viribus electricitatis in motu musculari commentarius* (Bologna: Ex typographia Instituti Scientiarum, 1791).
2. "The Science of Stretch," *The Scientist*, accessed October 1, 2017, https://www.the-scientist.com/features/the-science-of-stretch-39407.
3. H. M. Langevin, D. L. Churchill, and M. J. Cipolla, "Mechanical Signaling through Connective Tissue: A Mechanism for the Therapeutic Effect of Acupuncture," *FASEB Journal* 15, no. 12 (2001): 2275–82.
4. Ibid.
5. H. M. Langevin et al., "Biomechanical Response to Acupuncture Needling in Humans," *Journal of Applied Physiology* 91, no. 6 (2001): 2471–78.
6. http://www.biologyreference.com/Ce-Co/Connective-Tissue.html.
7. James Reston, "Now, About My Operation in Peking," *The New York Times*, July 26, 1971, https://www.nytimes.com/1971/07/26/archives/now-about-my-operation-in-peking-now-let-me-tell-you-about-my.html.
8. Ibid.
9. "NCCIH Facts-at-a-Glance and Mission," The National Center for Complementary and Integrative Health, accessed January 1, 2018, https://nccih.nih.gov/about/ataglance.

10. "Needles and Coffee May Not Mix; Even a Low Dose of Caffeine Blocks Acupuncture's Pain Relief in Mice," The National Center for Complementary and Integrative Health, accessed January 1, 2018, https://nccih .nih.gov/research/results/spotlight/needles-coffee.

11. Dominic P. Lu, D.D.S. and Gabriel P. Lu, "An Historical Review and Perspective on the Impact of Acupuncture," *Medical Acupuncture* 25, no. 5 (2013): 311–16.

12. D. Colquhoun and S. P. Novella, "Acupuncture Is Theatrical Placebo," *Anesthesia & Analgesia* 116, no. 6 (2013): 1360–63.

13. S. Takayama et al., "Evaluation of the Effects of Acupuncture on Blood Flow in Humans with Ultrasound Color Doppler Imaging," *Evidence-Based Complementary and Alternative Medicine* (2012).

14. D. W. Spence et al., "Acupuncture Increases Nocturnal Melatonin Secretion and Reduces Insomnia and Anxiety: A Preliminary Report," *Journal of Neuropsychiatry and Clinical Neurosciences* 16, no. 1 (2004): 19–28.

15. S. Hua et al., "Effects of Electroacupuncture on Depression and the Production of Glial Cell Line–Derived Neurotrophic Factor Compared with Fluoxetine: A Randomized Controlled Pilot Study," *Journal of Alternative and Complementary Medicine* 19, no. 9 (2013): 733–39.

16. C. H. Peng, M. M. Yang, S. H. Kok, and Y. K. Woo, "Endorphin Release: A Possible Mechanism of Acupuncture Analgesia," *American Journal of Chinese Medicine* 6, no. 1 (1978): 57–60.

17. J. N. Kenyon, C. J. Knight, and C. Wells, "Randomized Double-Blind Trial on the Immediate Effects of Naloxone on Classical Chinese Acupuncture Therapy for Chronic Pain," *Acupuncture & Electro-Therapeutics Research* 8, no. 1 (1983): 17–24.

18. C. R. Chapman, C. Benedetti, Y. H. Colpitts, and R. Gerlach, "Naloxone Fails to Reverse Pain Thresholds Elevated by Acupuncture: Acupuncture Analgesia Reconsidered," *Pain* 16, no. 1 (1983): 13–31.

19. Markham Heid, "Does Acupuncture Work?" *TIME*, June 29, 2016, http://time.com/4383611/acupuncture-alternative-medicine-pain/.

20. Ibid.

21. Ming Qing Zhu and Moyee Siu, "Can Acupuncture Really Benefit Stroke Recovery?" Pacific College of Oriental Medicine, https://www .pacificcollege.edu/news/blog/2015/07/27/can-acupuncture-really-benefit -stroke-recovery.

22. D. Keown, *The Spark in the Machine: How the Science of Acupuncture Explains the Mysteries of Western Medicine* (London: Singing Dragon Publishers, 2014).

23. Ibid., 50.

24. A. M. Turing, F.R.S., "The Chemical Basis of Morphogenesis," The Royal Society Publishing, August 14, 1952, DOI: 10.1098/rstb.1952.0012.

25. "CT Scans Reveal Acupuncture Points," HealthCMi, January 4, 2014, http://www.healthcmi.com/Acupuncture-Continuing-Education-News/1230-new-ct-scans-reveal-acupuncture-points.

26. Ibid.

27. A. Ovechkin, S. M. Lee, and K. S. Kim, "Thermovisual Evaluation of Acupuncture Points," *Acupuncture & Electro-Therapeutics Research*, 26, nos. 1–2 (2001): 11–23.

28. N. Tsuruoka, M. Watanabe, T. Seki, T. Matsunaga, and Y. Hagaa, "Acupoint Stimulation Device Using Focused Ultrasound," Conference Proceedings: IEEE Engineering in Medicine and Biology Annual Conference (2010): 1258–61.

29. D. Keown, *The Spark in the Machine: How the Science of Acupuncture Explains the Mysteries of Western Medicine* (London: Singing Dragon Publishers, 2014).

30. C. Shang, "Prospective Tests on Biological Models of Acupuncture," *Evidence-Based Complementary and Alternative Medicine* 6, no. 1 (2009): 31–39.

31. C. Shang, "Electrophysiology of Growth Control and Acupuncture," *Life Science* 68, no. 12 (2001):1333–42.

32. D. Keown, *The Spark in the Machine: How the Science of Acupuncture Explains the Mysteries of Western Medicine* (London: Singing Dragon Publishers, 2014), 77.

33. T. W. Findley, "Fascia Research from a Clinician/Scientist's Perspective," *International Journal of Therapeutic Massage & Bodywork* 4, no. 4 (2011): 1–6.

34. Ibid., 79.

35. Ibid., 85.

36. D. Church and D. Feinstein, "Manual Stimulation of Acupuncture Points in the Treatment of Post-Traumatic Stress Disorder: A Review of Clinical Emotional Freedom Techniques," *Medical Acupuncture* 29, no. 4 (2017): 194–205.

37. Tufts University, https://www.youtube.com/watch?v=ndFe5CaDTlI.

38. Tufts Now, http://now.tufts.edu/news-releases/face-frog-time-lapse-video-reveals-never-seen.

39. Daniel Keown, in discussion with the author, February 2017.

Chapter 6: Hands-On Activities

1. L. Katerina and T. Cynthia, "The Regulation of the Practice of Acupuncture by Physicians in the United States," *Medical Acupuncture* 29, no. 3 (2017): 121–27.

2. M. Eliade, *Shamanism: Archaic Techniques of Ecstasy* (Princeton: The Princeton/Bollingen Series in World Mythology, 2004).

3. Carla Kreft, in discussion with the author.

4. Ibid.

5. Ibid.

6. Ibid.

7. Ibid.

8. Ibid.

9. Ibid.

10. Ibid.

11. Ibid.

12. "Andrew Bassett, Orthopedist, Is Dead at 70," *Columbia University Record*, Volume 20, Columbia University, accessed, February 3rd 2018, http://www.columbia.edu/cu/record/archives/vol20/vol20_iss12/record 2012.34.html.

13. See Chapter 4.

14. A. Seto et al., "Detection of Extraordinary Large Bio-Magnetic Field Strength from Human Hand During External Qi Emission," *Acupuncture & Electro-Therapeutics Research* 17, no. 2 (1992): 75–94.

15. C. Andrew L. Bassett, "Beneficial Effects of Electromagnetic Fields," *Journal of Cellular Biochemistry* 51 (1993): 387–93.

16. *Columbia University Record*, Volume 20, Columbia University, accessed September 1, 2017, http://www.columbia.edu/cu/record/archives/vol20/vol20_iss12/record2012.34.html.

17. James L. Oschman, *Energy Medicine: The Scientific Basis* (New York: Elsevier Ltd., 2016).

18. Ibid., 250.

19. Bernadette Doran, BS, RMT, "The Science Behind Reiki," https://www.equilibrium-e3.com/images/PDF/Science%20Behind%20Reiki.pdf.

20. Further evidence of this is documented in "The Electricity of Touch" by the HeartMath Institute.
21. Erik Peper, in discussion with the author, January 2018.
22. Ibid.
23. Ibid.
24. Ibid.

Chapter 7: Mystics Among Us

1. The publication ceased operations in 1986, and an online edition of this (unfortunately) does not exist.
2. Mitsumasa Kawakami, in discussion with the author, November 2017.
3. Erik Peper, in discussion with the author, 2017.
4. P. Arambula, E. Peper, M. Kawakami, and K. Hughes Gibney, "The Physiological Correlates of Kundalini Yoga Meditation: A Study of a Yoga Master," *Applied Psychophysiology and Biofeedback* 26, no. 2 (2001): 147–53.
5. Erik Peper, in discussion with the author.
6. Leah Lagos, in discussion with the author.
7. Erik Peper, in discussion with the author, 2017.
8. Kevin Gray, "Inside Silicon Valley's New Non-Religion: Consciousness Hacking," November 1, 2017, https://www.wired.co.uk/article/consciousness-hacking-silicon-valley-enlightenment-brain.
9. J. Riba, S. Romero, E. Grasa, E. Mena, I. Carrió, and M. J. Barbanoj, "Increased Frontal and Paralimbic Activation Following Ayahuasca, the Pan-Amazonian Inebriant," *Psychopharmacology* 186, no. 1 (2006): 93–98.
10. Nell Casey, "Just Don't Mention Timothy Leary," *Whole Health Report*, http://www.nellcaseywriter.com/pdfs/psych.pdf.
11. C. S. Grob, A. L. Danforth, G. S. Chopra, M. Hagerty, C. R. McKay, A. L Halberstadt, and G. R. Greer, "Pilot Study of Psilocybin Treatment for Anxiety in Patients with Advanced-stage Cancer," *Archives of General Psychiatry* 68, no. 1 (2011): 71–78.
12. R. R. Griffiths, W. A. Richards, U. McCann, and R. Jesse, "Psilocybin Can Occasion Mystical-Type Experiences Having Substantial and Sustained Personal Meaning and Spiritual Significance," *Psychopharmacology* 187, no. 3 (2006).
13. R. R. Griffiths, W. A. Richards, M. W. Johnson, U. D. McCann, and R. Jesse, "Mystical-Type Experiences Occasioned by Psilocybin Mediate

the Attribution of Personal Meaning and Spiritual Significance 14 Months Later," *Psychopharmacology* 22, no. 6 (2008): 621–32.

14. R. R. Griffiths, M. W. Johnson, W. A. Richards, B. D. Richards, U. McCann, and R. Jesse, "Psilocybin Occasioned Mystical-Type Experiences: Immediate and Persisting Dose-Related Effects," *Psychopharmacology* 218, no. 4 (2011): 649–65.

15. R. L. Carhart-Harris, "Neural Correlates of the LSD Experience Revealed by Multimodal Neuroimaging," *PNAS* 113, no. 17 (2016): 4853–58.

16. Ibid.

17. Erik Peper, in discussion with the author, 2017.

Chapter 8: What's in a Placebo?

1. M. Spencer, "The Power of Nothing: Could Studying the Placebo Effect Change the Way We Think about Medicine?" *The New Yorker*, December 12, 2011, https://www.newyorker.com/magazine/2011/12/12 /the-power-of-nothing.

2. Ibid.

3. Ibid.

4. Ibid.

5. H. K. Beecher, "The Powerful Placebo," *Journal of the American Medical Association* 159, no. 17 (1955):1602–6.

6. F. Benedetti et al., "Teaching Neurons to Respond to Placebos," *Journal of Physiology* 594, no. 19 (2016): 5647–60.

7. R. Klinger, M. Blasini, J. Schmitz, and L. Colloca, "Nocebo Effects in Clinical Studies: Hints for Pain Therapy," *Pain Reports* 2, no. 2 (2017).

8. Ibid.

9. M. Spencer, "The Power of Nothing: Could Studying the Placebo Effect Change the Way We Think about Medicine?" *The New Yorker*, December 12, 2011, https://www.newyorker.com/magazine/2011/12/12 /the-power-of-nothing.

10. J. Kong et al., "A Functional Magnetic Resonance Imaging Study on the Neural Mechanisms of Hyperalgesic Nocebo Effect," *Journal of Neuroscience* 28, no. 49 (2008): 13354—62; J. Kong et al., "Brain Activity Associated with Expectancy-Enhanced Placebo Analgesia as Measured by Functional Magnetic Resonance Imaging," *Journal of Neuroscience* 26, no. 2 (2006): 381–88; T. J. Kaptchuk, P. Goldman, D. A. Stone, and

W. B. Stason, "Do Medical Devices Have Enhanced Placebo Effects?" *Journal of Clinical Epidemiology* 53 (2000): 786–92.

11. T. J. Kaptchuk et al., "Components of Placebo Effect: Randomized Controlled Trial in Patients with Irritable Bowel Syndrome," *British Medical Journal* 332 (2006): 391–97.

12. Ibid.

13. Ian Harris, *Surgery, the Ultimate Placebo: A Surgeon Cuts Through the Evidence* (Sydney: NewSouth Publishing, 2016), Kindle location 2309.

14. Ted Kaptchuk, in discussion with the author.

15. Ian Harris, *Surgery, the Ultimate Placebo: A Surgeon Cuts Through the Evidence* (Sydney: NewSouth Publishing, 2016).

16. Dr. Ian Harris, in discussion with the author, October 2017.

17. Ibid.

18. Richard Deyo, "Epidemiology of Spinal Surgery: Rates and Trends," School of Public Health, University of Washington, http://depts .washington.edu/ccor/studies/SpineSurgEpi.shtml; J. T. Street et al., "Morbidity and Mortality of Major Adult Spinal Surgery: A Prospective Cohort Analysis of 942 Consecutive Patients," *Spine Journal* 12, no. 1 (2012): 22–34; A. J. Schoenfeld, L. M. Ochoa, J. O. Bader, P. J. Belmont Jr., "Risk Factors for Immediate Postoperative Complications and Mortality Following Spine Surgery: A Study of 3475 Patients from the National Surgical Quality Improvement Program," *Journal of Bone and Joint Surgery* (American) 3, no. 17 (2011): 1577–82; Richard Deyo et al., "Trends, Major Medical Complications, and Charges Associated with Surgery for Lumbar Spinal Stenosis in Older Adults," *Journal of the American Medical Association* 303, no. 13 (2010):1259–65.

19. Dr. Ian Harris, in discussion with the author, October 2017.

20. Ian Harris, *Surgery, the Ultimate Placebo: A Surgeon Cuts Through the Evidence* (Sydney: NewSouth Publishing, 2016), Kindle locations 981–82.

21. Erik Peper, in discussion with the author.

22. Ibid.

23. C. Carvalho, J. M. Caetano, L. Cunha, P. Rebouta, T. J. Kaptchuk, and I. Kirsch, "Open-Label Placebo Treatment in Chronic Low Back Pain: A Randomized Controlled Trial," *Journal of Pain* (2016).

24. Reuters, "Placebos Help, Even When Patients Know About Them," https://www.reuters.com/article/us-placebo/placebos-help-even-when -patients-know-about-them-idUSTRE6BL4IU20101222.

25. A. H. Tuttle, S. Tohyama, T. Ramsay, J. Kimmelman, P. Schweinhardt, G. J. Bennett, J. S. Mogil, "Increasing Placebo Responses Over Time in U.S. Clinical Trials of Neuropathic Pain," *Pain* 156, no. 12 (2015): 2616–26.

26. Melissa Dahl, "The Placebo Effect Is Getting Stronger—But Only in the U.S.," *The Cut*, October 9, 2015, https://www.thecut.com/2015/10/placebo-effect-is-getting-stronger.html.

27. W. F. Bengston and M. Moga, "Resonance, Placebo Effects, and Type II Errors: Some Implications from Healing Research for Experimental Methods," *Journal of Alternative and Complementary Medicine* 13, no. 3 (2007): 317–27.

Chapter 9: You the Healer

1. Madhu Anziani, in discussion with the author.

2. Madhu Anziani, in discussion with the author.

3. "On the Meaning of: OM MANI PADME HUM," Sacred Texts, accessed January 21, 2017, http://www.sacred-texts.com/bud/tib/omph.htm.

4. Madhu Anziani, in discussion with the author.

5. Ibid.

6. Ibid.

7. Ibid.

8. B. G. Kalyani et al., "Neurohemodynamic Correlates of 'OM' Chanting: A Pilot Functional Magnetic Resonance Imaging Study," *International Journal of Yoga* 4, no. 1 (2011): 3–6.

9. C. Grape et al., "Does Singing Promote Well-Being?: An Empirical Study of Professional and Amateur Singers During a Singing Lesson," *Integrative Physiological and Behavioral Science* 38, no. 1 (2003): 65–74.

10. "Inside Stressing Out: What Works and What Doesn't in the Face of Stress," The Institute of HeartMath, https://www.heartmath.com/articles/inside-stressing-out-what-works-and-what-doesnt-in-the-face-of-stress/.

11. Ibid.

12. C. B. Pert, *Molecules of Emotion: The Science Behind Mind-Body Medicine* (New York: Simon & Schuster, 2010), e-book.

13. T. G. Gutheil and A. Brodsky, *Preventing Boundary Violations in Clinical Practice* (New York: Guilford Press, 2008).

14. Dr. Thomas Gutheil, in discussion with the author.

15. T. G. Gutheil and A. Brodsky, *Preventing Boundary Violations in Clinical Practice* (New York: Guilford Press, 2008), 30.

Chapter 10: Let There Be Light

1. M. Kobayashi, D. Kikuchi, and H. Okamura, "Imaging of Ultraweak Spontaneous Photon Emission from Human Body Displaying Diurnal Rhythm," *PLOS ONE* 4, no. 7 (2009): e6256, https://doi.org/10.1371/journal.pone.0006256.
2. F. A. Popp, "MO-Rechnungen an 3,4-Benzpyren und 1,2-Benzpyren legen ein Mod-ell zur Deutung der chemischen Karzinogenese nahe," *Zeitschrift für Natur-forschung* 27b (1972): 731; F. A. Popp, "Einige Möglichkeiten für Biosignale zur Steuerung des Zellwachstums," *Archiv für Geschwulstforschung* 44 (1974): 295–306.
3. Ibid.
4. "Dr. Fritz-Albert Popp Thought He Had Discovered a Cure for Cancer," Biontology Arizona, https://www.biontologyarizona.com/fritz-albert-popp-cure-for-cancer/.
5. L. McTaggart, *The Field—The Quest for the Secret Force of the Universe* (New York: HarperCollins Publishers, 2008), 53.
6. Kiran Trace, in discussion with the author, February 2018, New York.

INDEX

ABOUT THE AUTHOR

JILL BLAKEWAY holds a doctorate in acupuncture and Chinese medicine and is a licensed and board certified acupuncturist and clinical herbalist. She is known for the intuitive way she practices Chinese medicine and for her ability to integrate this ancient practice with modern biomedicine. Jill is the founder of the Yinova Center in New York City. She is also a visiting professor of traditional Chinese medicine at Pacific College of Oriental Medicine, where she offers a course on gynecology and obstetrics for doctoral candidates. Jill is the coauthor of Making Babies and the author of Sex Again.